C O P I N G
A N D
B E Y O N D

Being
A Surgeon's Reflections
on
Medicine, Science, Art
and
A Life Worth Living

MONEIM A. FADALI, M.D.

DeVorss & Company, Publishers

ISBN: 0-87516-621-0
Library of Congress Catalog Card Number: 89-80976

Third Printing, 1999

DeVorss & Company, Publisher
P.O. Box 550
Marina del Rey, CA 90294

Printed in The United States of America

To

Homo sapiens

Struggling to learn, when all
you must do is remember.

> —American Indian poem

I alone know what I can do.
To others I am only a "perhaps."

> —Stendhal

Contents

PART TWO
On Being Creative and Free

Preface

I traveled, I wandered, I never left my birthplace
and I long for the city of light.
—Author's poem "Questioning"

I DON'T CONSIDER this work a book in the customary sense. It is rather an experience transformed into words. A voice long silent has at last chosen to sound. Lacking the talent to paint an inferno or a paradise, let alone a seagull or a child; devoid of the sculptor's touch—my statues remain uncut, buried in a quarry somewhere—and without Orpheus' lyre; I have had to rest my case in words—all despite the realization that in attempting to express the inexpressible, words get in the way and a measure of injustice is bound to happen. A predicament for which I have no cure. While attempting to fix his heroine Emma Bovary to the page, Gustave Flaubert wrote, "Language is like a cracked kettle on which we beat our tunes for bears to dance to; while all the time we long to move the stars to pity." Pen in hand and counting on your discretion, I take on the risk of telling you what I know of myself and what I have seen, what is "going on," and what I hope for. Deep inside me a medieval troubadour pulls the strings and beats the drum. We travel together.

Ever since I can remember—age five, six, seven, perhaps—I have been writing in my mind and living my lines. It all began as I sat in the shade of an old, old sycamore tree gazing into the sky, witnessing sunrise, waiting for sunset, and talking to the moon. The wind in the reeds and the soothing sound of water flowing in an unnamed winding creek kept me company. Here songbirds come and go, trilling, quibbling over who knows what. Herds of sheep, cows, buffalo and guard dogs pass me by. Down-to-earth peasants and shepherds hurry in the faint dawn light, some mounted on the backs of their patient donkeys.

Morning air—fresh, gentle, kind, bringing aromas of orange blossoms, peppermint, and jasmine. Moments before dusk, the same procession returns, heading in the opposite direction. Tired men dragging their heavy feet, singing solo, or in chorus, rhymes of toil, deferred hope, submission to fate, the life of one day at a time and contentment with simple things. At times a flute, a *mizmar*, tablas, or tambourines will join in, adding sweet melody to an otherwise somber scene.

I have always paid fond attention to farm animals. To this day my mind's eye clearly sees their sad, dark eyes turning toward me. I still recall and refeel the stabs of pain and waves of sorrow their melancholy gaze has given me. In stark contrast: the affability and jollity of farm dogs, tirelessly wagging happy tails, affectionately displaying their tongues, instantly transformed into what seems a big smile.

Again, the old, old tree, the sky, the sun, the birds, the reeds, the herd, dogs, peasants, shepherds, other things—myself included—all reflected in the same water, all fitted into the scheme of life, all subject to transiency and destined to be variously consumed. And of these, some are set in a relation of conflict. The apparent contending forces of opposition, inexplicable and for the most part disturbing, must have weighed heavily on my mind.

Perhaps to resolve the unsettling matter or to escape from it, I reflexly threw stones in the water, conveniently breaking these images of opposition. At that time, such a lofty interpretation of my behavior would never have crossed my mind; it was all rather spontaneous. Now the rationalizing adult is looking back, exploring the former child. And both happen to be me.

Letting memory speak, I can recall my very first wish; my first heartache; the wholehearted laughter of my childhood; those uncertain steps of mine as I began plowing—and experiencing different things, some labeled good, some bad; my fears; my early frustrations; and tears that burnt my cheeks, and their salty taste; my timid, secret yearning for love; my dancing, happy heart as I fell in love; and my heavy heart when I fell out of love; my mysterious inner experiences with God, religion, doubt and belief; happiness' first embrace; maiden perceptions of danger; scars; loneliness and loss; and songs once heard, never to leave my heart, to this very day.

Drifting along, I took the long step from Tizmant to Los Angeles—"L.A.," where the river meets the ocean. A city within a city, a city of deflowered innocence, church bells, chimes, tall banks, flotation tanks, Mickey Mouse, drugs, punks, rockers, and restless adolescence. A city opening its arms to the rich, the famous, the drifter, the wanderer, and the reborn artist. A city of long boulevards, short shady alleys, bougainvillea, oleanders, jacarandas, palm trees, birds of paradise, "cruisemobiles," smog, laser beams and candlelight. L.A.: a state of mind.

The journey took many years. On the road, destiny and design took me to small and big towns and to countries with differing land, weather, customs, religion, and tongue. A mosaic, intriguing and utterly splendid. On the surface dissimilar, at times mutually repulsive, yet their true essence was one of resemblance and harmony. An amazing web spun from threads of all kinds of elements, colors, and temperaments. Any nation, mighty or meek, is merely a strand of the web; and whatever it chooses to do to the web it does to itself. I took time studying, working, visiting, and simply loafing. As I entered the shallows of life, the shadow of my old, old sycamore tree moved farther and farther from me; yet the scene never faded away, and its script remained legible. Tizmant, the remote dusty village by the sycamore tree, remained the capital of my mind. Its gravitational field can still pull me—and I know it. Whenever the east wind blows balmy and loving, I see the tree and hear the creek calling my name.

Moving along, I encountered trees older and taller than myself, with tales to tell; and I listened somewhat—not enough, though; not enough. Was I in a hurry? Still, I would stop to take note of a lonely yellow dandelion making it through the asphalt pavement of a busy city street; grass sprouts bursting through concrete; a blind man reciting a poem; the eager hands of deaf children touching the stage while the band was playing; a young woman paralyzed from her waist down selling flowers in a town square; a Hiroshima survivor who lost the basic features of her face, enthusiastically—without hate or malice—recounting the great horror to a huge rally for nuclear disarmament and world peace; an excommunicated priest taking his sermon to the road; an old man climbing 37 steps to water his vegetable patch; an old woman with aching legs walking her old dog in the park on a dreary winter day; lizards gallivanting in the scorching desert; a parched tree trunk, rejuvenated by unexpected rain, letting out new branches and pretty green leaves; heavy fog lifting off the pier. The message: *Hang On.*

And on this journey I met abandoned dogs; starving coyotes; acid rain; dead lakes and poisoned fishes; seagulls unable to fly; plumeless birds; barren forests; children of affluence on merry-go-rounds, others raised to starve, beg, and suffer; poets cold and indifferent, others gusting with passion; writers sold out, transfigured into cackling parrots and silly clowns; others eagerly holding on to their pens, articulating humanity's cause and high mission; scientists intent on hiding the sun and adulterating the air, recklessly inventing hideous tools for sons of Cain to annihilate the near and the far, ever so swiftly; others ardently working for the preservation of life and improving the human condition; reformers and free-thinkers silenced and muzzled; members of the clergy eroding their bellies while groveling in the dust before worldly authority, shamelessly blessing the rifle and the bomb, dispensing hypocrisy for religion, peddling seats in heaven for those whose purse could afford the price; politicians with platform eloquence, infatuated with power, steeped in greed, waging war to end war, their souls consumed by a ghastly fire. What was left? Dancing silhouettes named *deception*; ashes called *intrigue.*

I heard someone singing, "If it ain't for bad luck, I won't have any luck at all." This wrenched my heart. Someone else rejoiced, "What a wonderful day!" This gave me hope and a smile. A third chanted, "Raindrops keep falling on my head, but that does not mean my eyes will soon be turning red." This conveyed a sense of reality and a measure of relief. You see, I take my songs seriously; and may I say: if you want to look into a nation's soul, open its book of songs.

On a carrousel horse, a flying carpet, a treadmill, a roller-coaster, within a labyrinth nicknamed ego, along the seekers' trail and on the path of the believers: I saw the holy and the profane, the rational and the intuitive, the realist and the dreamer, the sane and the insane, the elite and the vulgar, the confident and the conceited, the wise and the fool—all in pursuit of paradise.

What, then, has come of it all? It isn't for me to tell. Can't find my tongue.

The pages of this book began, and for the most part continued, as an accumulation of seeming odds and ends, driven by a force of their own. Notes scribbled on scrap-paper for no better reason than self-expression, footnotes entered on book pages while reading them, letters to friends, chit-chats with individuals met on purpose and by accident. People—just people—all kinds; a fascinating spectrum arbitrarily classified by our social yard-sticks into the good and the bad, the high and the low—criteria I find wanting, ambiguous, and for the most part biased if not outright ridiculous and malicious.

In putting the material together, one strand recurs throughout, an axis best defined as a timely desire to see clearly, and to rip off an imaginary—but in effect an actual—mask standing between the eye of my mind and reality. All I did was scratch different stations of my mind, with editing consciously kept to a minimum, for the most part to follow rules of grammar or to relocate certain pieces gone astray, yet belonging to and complementing one another.

I am fully aware that even the unreferenced portions of this book cannot be exclusively mine. As we move about, certain actions, thoughts, and words of others stay on and for one reason or another lay hold of us. As time goes on, certain of these gravitate into our private interiors, where they are no more perceived as alien. In this sense, no work of art or literature is truly original. Only the boastful and the vain claim utter originality.

Now, after due consideration, the time has come. My book is full, complete; all I need do is lay it open and let its pages unfold one after the other. If you choose to read it through, I hope it will hold meaning for you. And if any part—even a tiny fragment, a line, a short phrase, or a mere passing thought—touches your heart, this will be my great joy, for in reaching you, I will be realizing my own existence and finding another part of my true worth.

COPING
AND
BEYOND

PART ONE
ON RIGHT SEEING

Straightforward words seem paradoxical.
                              —Tao Te Ching

I'd rather be able to see.
 —Martin in John Osborne's play *Luther*

Don't think: Look.
                              —Ludwig Wittgenstein

The Time Is at Hand

HAPPY BIRTHDAY TO YOU, HAPPY BIRTHDAY TO YOU! The band plays, the crowd hails, and everyone sings; finally, a certain number of flickering candles are blown out and everybody gets a piece of the cake. Happiness fills the air and everyone toasts the good time. All looks splendid. But when the party is over, the aftertaste isn't always sweet and happy. A remote sense of melancholy and a measure of panic often sneak in. Unsettling questions often arise: "What have I accomplished so far? Wasted my years; and life is too short. Time takes it away. Where do I go from here? God! If only I could know!"

I know of some acquaintances and friends who have stopped celebrating their birthdays altogether. The party, with all its cake, candlelight, and music, echoes the ticking sound of a timer forecasting the inevitable—a requiem for yesteryear, accentuating loss and underscoring the diminishing reserves.

As far as I am concerned: I couldn't care less how old I am. Every day is my birthday. I can't stop the perpetual passing of time, and if I could—and did—I'd be doing myself in. Time's perpetual motion is an integral manifestation of life. If time ever did stand still, surely I'd be stilled with it. I can't turn the clock back for a refund, so I'd better befriend time and travel with it hand in hand, with no pushing, no pulling, no quarrels —and no remorse for hours and days gone by.

In the realm of the present, I am merely a child, as young as a rosebud and ever will be: a child of the present. In the realm of the past, I am as old as the hills, many thousand years old, and within me are the experiences of thousands of men, women, and children. Anticipating the future, I am hoping, ever renewing, resurrected time after time. So what difference does it make how old I am? How old are you?

Time's three dimensions form a continuum through which I travel and wander. Every moment is grand—full of wonder, opportunity, uniqueness, and excitement. Every time I open my eyes a little, I am amazed how much is left undone and how much needs to be done.

Every morning as your unwilling feet drag you over to the bathroom, where you meet your grumbling face in the mirror, lay down your toothbrush and wish yourself a Happy Birthday. Any day, every day, and all days: you are resurrected, renewed, given power and new opportunities. Any time, any season, any year, you can do what you ought and want to do. Be good to yourself; smile; your smile will cheer your countenance and brighten your outlook. *You* are the keeper of the "clock." So fuss no more; waste no more. Joy to you! Joy to the world!

We are merely travelers in transit; we are not permanent dwellers in this corner of the Universe. Reviewing the history of humankind and the cosmos, my life—short or long as it may be—shrinks into a very brief moment, an almost trivial incident in the countless pages of eternity. Hindu astronomers, intrigued, called the cosmic cycles *kalpas*, and according to their calculations, one kalpa exceeds 4 billion years—mind-boggling, and perhaps an eye-opener.

Such considerations should compel our attention and focus it on our egocentric landscape, where we see but ourselves, solo without others—and apart from the Universe, its mountains, oceans, pastures, rivers, galaxies, solar systems, and—don't forget—the trees and the flowers, besides all else that grows, walks, creeps, and flies.

I consider myself fortunate, then, having made it thus far, and I can't just wipe out somber areas in my memory, areas populated by those who departed earlier on and who happened to be chronologically younger than myself. Some were unusually gifted, tender and throbbing with the vital force of life; more deserving, I thought, to live and linger longer. For sure, these kinds of "decisions" are not up to us. So I digress, I see, and am beginning to feel sad. Time to shift gears. Here we are: *alive*; and since we are alive, we had better attend to *life*. As part of the enterprise of life, this very hour calls for *looking*.

Looking: Where?

THE SPECTRUM: OCEANWIDE DIMENSIONS. INFINITE, the six directions diverge: east and west, north and south, high and low, time and space—all coexist without displacing one another. Ludwig Wittgenstein cautioned, "Don't think: look." In their solitude, pious souls implore, "Lord, that we might see!" Besieged and tormented, Martin Luther pleaded, "I'd rather be able to see."[1]

Let us ride on the wings of time. Where to? Does it matter? Since we habitually cling to *whereabouts*—and besides, we promised to travel together—therefore, wherever we are—on board ship ready for the sea; on an airplane, cruising above the clouds; on a train ride; on a lofty mountain peak; by the church's altar; in the limitless confines of a sacred temple; in a smoke-filled cafe; in the rat-race of the market place; alone or with a hundred others; anywhere—let's loose our tired frame, and let our programmed, pinioned mind go free. Its unshaded eye will soon be able to see.

Sunrise, sunset; moonlit and pitch-dark nights; seasons, calendars, clocks; birth, death, growth, decay; tales, library archives; unpaid old debts—all conspire in one form or another to fracture time's continuity and freeze its natural fluidity. With a little help from historians, analysts, and futurists, past, present, and future have become separate entities, each acquiring its own school and company of scholars.

Caught in the shadowy corridors of the past, our memory reproduces its good and its bad, not always free from errors of omission and commission. Human memory is notoriously selective, picky, with likes and dislikes, attractions and distractions, securities and liabilities—the whole works! Out of

1. *Luther*, a play by John Osborne (New York: New American Library, Signet Books, 1963), p. 51.

mother's womb, life starts wounding us all. Our very first utterance is a cry, a loud cry! True, we are not all bruised to the same degree—some are hurt deeper and more often—still, let alone, wounds heal. Debris and scars are left behind, though habitually, from time to time, we can't help but touch our tender spots; after all, they are known to us, *we were there.* It is human to feel at home within one's past—more or less. Up to this point, we are all together; beyond, the trail branches off. After pausing for reflection, the prudent move on, while others idle and linger, and some dwell in their private caves, reviewing the old graffiti.

Clinging to the past—glorious, ordinary, or scandalous—will take us nowhere. Neither pride nor self-pity solves problems or heals injury. Pride blinds and corrupts, pity demoralizes and de-energizes—human-made alibis for self-praise, self-excuse, and blaming others. Pats on the back. *In the latitudes of the past, reflect when necessary; but the less, the better. Cling not, and if the train of thought takes you to Memory Land, fly back. The present waits for no one. Moment by moment it steadily moves to its own destination: the past.*

What about the future? Man habitually attaches himself to a pendulum swinging to and fro between past and future. The present becomes incidental, casually acknowledged in between swings. This is nothing new and comes to no one's surprise. Ever since man trod the surface of the earth, the future caught his eye and captured his imagination. Not without justification: formless, limitless, the future is perfectly suited to accommodate our aspirations and dreams. Its untried material readily lends itself to building castles, digging tunnels too. No sweat. No tears.

To voice complete disinterest in future matters repels credibility and is impractical. After all, hope—the indispensable elixir of the human spirit, the ship that carries us through the roughest times—can only materialize in the future. And of all the freedoms we have, hope is the only freedom no one can take away from us. As such, the future is a human asset, very precious.

8

However, setbacks befall us when the present is bartered away for the future. It's a bad deal on all counts—too much is given away for too little; perhaps something is exchanged for nothing at all. For we can exist only in the present. The past cannot be lived any more, save for memory. And the future is yet to come.

Sweet and full of longing, unreasonable dreams of rainbows to come constitute an adult disease that rarely afflicts children. Baited and lured by tomorrow, grown-ups forget to live. Within the eternal cycle, the future is born out of the present. It is taking shape right now, always at this very instant. This being so, at this moment let us shape the shapeless mass—*before it shapes us.*

Listen to the exhortation of the Dawn!
Look to this Day, for it is Life.
The very Life of Life.

In its brief course lie all the verities,
The realities of your existence:
The bliss of growth, the glory of action.
The splendor of beauty;

For yesterday is but a dream,
And tomorrow is only a vision;
But today, well lived,
Makes yesterday a dream of happiness
And every tomorrow a vision of hope.

Look well, therefore, to this Day!

—*The Salutation of the Dawn*

Questions and Answers:
The Puzzle and the Dilemma

EVERYWHERE WE LOOK WE ENCOUNTER THE FAMILIAR and the unfamiliar, the known and the unknown. Questions readily arise. As for the answers, some come easily enough, while others seem never to come; and most lie somewhere in between. Unanswered questions tend to repeat themselves, teasing the mind. A puzzle unsolved acts as a focus of irritation and a reason for discontent. Faced with the challenge, some keep looking for solutions, others give up, drifting through the familiar escape route; clutching at memories and trusting in dreams that will magically solve the puzzle and restore order to the troubled mind.

In order of time, answers actually come first, predating their respective questions. As a matter of fact, *answers generate their own questions*—not the other way around. We readily acknowledge the questions because they stare us in the face, dancing before our very eyes, challenging our wits, at times jolting our confidence and undermining our sense of security. Answers for the most part lie hidden beneath the rubbish or in unlikely corners, *some disguised as questions*. And it is meant to be that way, enhancing the game, making it more dynamic and interesting, besides sorting out who does his homework and who does not.

Thorough search with joyful contemplation and renewed will can solve any puzzle and open the door. The seeker seeks, and on coming up with the answer, he gleefully announces: I found it! Seeking and finding something that never existed is unrealistic. To the restless, questioning mind, it is reassuring to realize that for all our questions, *solutions preexist*, waiting to be uncovered. Questions that have no answers do not exist and never did.

The question/answer puzzle is a never-ending daily human affair. Right Seeing holds the key to unlocking the safe where some of our most valuable articles are deposited. At all times, wise men have been sought out by the elite and the crowd. They have the answers, so we believe. And frequently they do. They are called seers. The word *seer* derives from the verb *to see*. Wisdom means seeing. One qualification, though: it must be Right Seeing. An encouraging footnote: we do not have to travel very far to see aright.

> Not knowing how near the Truth is,
> People seek it far away—what a pity!
>
> —Hakuin's *Song of Meditation*[1]

1. Quoted in D. T. Suzuki, *Essays in Zen Buddhism, First Series* (New York: Grove Press, 1978), p. 336.

On Looking: Is There a Problem?
If So, What Is It?

ON LOOKING AROUND US, ARE WE TRULY SEEING what we are looking at? And how often do we see objects the way they really are? These questions sound absurd, irrelevant, and yet they are valid and worthy. It is a matter of habit that at the instant of seeing, our individual subjective feeling is automatically thrown into the picture, distorting the object we are looking at. All conforms with what we already know. As a result, the very object we are seeing is altered, ceasing to be what it really is.

With our own shadow cast upon our surroundings, our open eyes go blind; the moon eclipses, flowers wither, time and place become imperceptible and slip by. With our ears turning deaf, the nightingale's perpetual song grows silent and the ceaseless sound of the sea abruptly ends. The actual spectacle is erased and we are left alone, staring in the blankness, hostage to our point of view. No moon to relish, no flowers to enjoy, no birds to watch and admire; merely a train of wandering thoughts— reruns, worn-out scenarios, recycled from time to time, conveniently retouched.

On his way to the scaffold, John Brown stopped for a moment of reflection, looked around, and uttered his final words: "This is a very beautiful world; I never noticed it before!"

> Stars are the windows of Heaven
> That Angels peek through.
> When we are happy, they are happy;
> When we are blue, they turn blue.

> —Irving Berlin, "All Alone"

Al and "La Valentina":
A Spectacle of Sorrow

ON A WARM, STARRY NIGHT IN MAY, MY CAR DROVE
me to a small neighborhood cafe, informal and cozy. Albert,
the owner, liked to sing, and on that night he sang a favorite
of his—a sad song. My mood must have been somber and reflec-
tive. I can't recall the lyrics, save for a verse that lingered on.
Paraphrased, it goes simply like this: As I look to the moon,
I see only you.

Al is a gifted singer, and a believable performer as well. Sip-
ping my capuccino while listening to him, I beheld his facial
expression growing sad, his tenor voice exuding melancholy.
It all bore an air of the genuine and the real. Poor Al, wasting
the moon! By his own admission, the world's magnificence and
splendor transforms into a fairy princess, the illusive sovereign
of his dreams. To what end?

Leaning on a forgotten elbow, with the blue rhymes and
rhythms charging the air, I began to experience some of my own
unexpressed sorrow—and somewhere in the backroads of my
mind an anonymous throat started singing "La Valentina"—a
song of sad commentary, perhaps a friendly testimonial sym-
pathetic to Al, or a timely echo reaffirming the tragic fate of
the haunted and the obsessed.[1]

> Because of my passion they say
> That ill fortune is on my way;
> It doesn't matter
> That it might be the devil himself.

---

1. It did happen; some time in 1987 tragedy struck, unexpected, ugly and
cruel. Someone shot Al, and this good soul died at the scene, relatively young,
say in his mid-fifties. Since then, I could not bring myself to go to this cafe
that I used to like. Al's death closed the place for me.

13

I do know how to die.
Valentina, Valentina,
I throw myself in your way.
If I am going to die tomorrow—
Why not once and for all today.

The whole story with its sad lyrics and seemingly unhappy characters retells the mournings and lamentations of many who are caught in similar straits. Their songs aren't all fiction, their sardonic dark verses betray real internal misery and, not uncommonly, a tragic state of mind. Juliet detested the lark; her agony still lives in verse and haunts the love story of many.

To all who are hurting while experiencing the downside of things: it is high time for new living arrangements. An upbeat song is worth considering, one with a happy ending. Suffering shouldn't be taken for a finale—it needn't be. Let it be merely an anguished chapter in the book of humankind. Life is an eventful play, and there isn't a memorable one without the painful scenes of tragedy. Continued suffering is uncalled-for; there is no good reason on earth for anyone to be cheated out of the simple joys and natural freedoms of life. According to Pascal, those of us who deserve commendation are those who manage to combine properly the sense of man's grandeur with a sense of his misery.

Right Seeing: What Is Standing in Our Way?

FOR RIGHT SEEING, WHERE SHALL WE GO? WHERE shall we look? Up to the high heavens and the stars above—or down to earth and her creatures? Shall we gaze into mirrors or down the highways that stretch ahead? Is it our *inside* that needs to be cracked and scrutinized? Shall we take refuge in prayers and rituals? What about contrition or repentance for what we have done or left undone? Would contemplation do it for us? Or should we sit still and *let* it happen? Alternatives interesting and not altogether devoid of merit; still, the bottom line is that, as a member of the human race, each of us is equipped with five senses and a mind that can interpret and discriminate. Having all these resources, where, then, shall we go from here?

> Each is given a bag
> of tools,
> A shapeless mass,
> A book of rules;
> And each must make
> —Ere life is flown—
> A stumbling block
> Or a stepping stone.
>
> —R. L. Sharpe

The stumbling block between us and right seeing is not an external one. It lies within and it happens to be our own intellect, always standing in the way, interpreting and explaining. All along, believing we are *seeing*, yet, by virtue of the

15

intellect we are *conceiving*. Seeing and conceiving are not synonymous; they differ substantially. In conceiving, objects are uniformly fertilized with our seeds of knowledge, expectation, apprehension, affection and disdain. The offspring is not going to be a copy of the original object! Consequently, *different* things come before us for judgment—the way we figure them out, the way we conceive them, the way we *think* they are—not the way they *are*.

Millennium after millennium, within the intriguing realm of the human mind, the speculative replaces the actual, the false substitutes for the true, the spurious is taken for the authentic and the fictitious for the genuine. As a result, the real world tumbles down and we find ourselves in a mock world, one of our own making and doing.

Among us, children and the wise see what they are looking at *as such*. This is the moral of the story "The Emperor's New Clothes." The Emperor rode naked and his procession passed through the streets. Only a child proclaimed him to be naked, while the rest of his subjects believed, from what they already "knew," that he was wearing his royal robes. Most of us must have heard the story before, but its brevity and precise message make it compelling and worth retelling.

Calling for Right Seeing while pointing an accusing finger at the intellect seems paradoxical and a bit disturbing. Are we thereby censoring the intellect? Are we condoning ignorance? Are we inviting unrestrained passion to rule our lives? Certainly not. And we'd better be not! We can't do without intellect, so let us put it right where it belongs—a stepping stone, not a stumbling block.

But permitting it to become a barrier between ourselves and the universe is absurd and foolhardy. Allowing it to disguise our true, higher Self beyond our recognition is shortsighted and tragic. Intellect, with its budding thought and blooming ideas, indispensable to humankind, must not be granted liberty to overtake the whole individual and override or undermine the will.

Self-mastery, the hallmark of good men and women, is attainable only if the will is freed to exercise its options and manifest its inexhaustible power. Once this comes to be, inner peace will follow—a free state of awareness with concord, mastery with harmony and sobriety. The enterprise is open to everyone, with no preconditions, no prior selections. All limitations, all exclusions are self-imagined, self-imposed.

Each Makes His Own World:
How Does This Come About?

KATSUKI SEKIDA, A RESPECTED ZEN TEACHER, SAYS, "The world in which each one of us finds himself is of his own making." In this connection, Buddhists teach that the eighteen elements of all our experience are: the six sense organs (eye, ear, nose, tongue, body, and mind); the six corresponding sense objects (forms, sounds, smells, tastes, touches, and objects of mind); and the six corresponding kinds of consciousness.

The five sense organs with which we customarily associate the senses define our "limits"—what belongs to us and what not; what constitutes our personhood. Things I see, hear, smell, taste or touch exist for *me*; I can recognize and acknowledge, choose to respond or ignore, and, if respond, decide what sort of response to make. Every day sunrays meet my eyes, stimulating minute receptors in my retinas; tiny electric waves are generated that travel along specialized nerve routes, finally reaching a specific area of my brain—the visual center. Then and there I see sunlight. In reality, my eyes *make* sunlight, and in one second they can process twenty-five images for me to view and scrutinize. Sunrays fall on plants and other living things lacking a visual system like ours. As far as we know, they do not produce visible light the way we do. The blind cannot make (see) sunlight, while anyone with intact eyesight may switch off the sun's illumination by drawing the eyelids together.

This unique system has three components: an object, a specialized sense organ, and a specific area in the brain. By similar processes my ears make the sound of the surf, music, and conversation by the cozy fireside; my nose prepares the rose's pleasing perfume; my tongue gathers the sweetness of honey and the bitterness of lime; and my palms bring forth the silky and the prickly. If my five senses decline or fail to process the myriads of stimuli they constantly receive, my brain will be out of work, left in limbo with nothing to do. Forms, sounds, smells, tastes, and touches will not find me. Instead, I shall be occupying a state of siege akin to hibernation or a hermetic isolation in which my existence will effectively cease. Sense organs deliver the world to us; in essence they make our world, they are our world.

Our Sense Organs: Perfectly Unbiased and Unique—Enjoying Health, They Are Completely Unaware of Themselves

A HEALTHY EYE CANNOT SEE ITSELF. DISEASED, IT will. In its state of self-awareness, we in turn become aware of it and seek a remedy. An ear that is well does not hear itself. Unhealthy, it will hear tinnitus—its own plea for help. The same goes for other organs of sense: only an unwell nose smells its own scent; an indisposed tongue will taste its gustation; and organs of touch, injured or ill, will experience a barrage of sense impressions even though untouched. Being self-detached, they are entirely free of bias, functioning as our faithful antennas, intercepting the world's folly and splendor just as they are. We, of course, are free to "take it or leave it."

Sense organs possess still another unique quality: they can't be coaxed or forced the way our voluntary muscles can. True, we have the option not to put them to work; but if we do, we are unable to entice them to fetch for us those particular sensations we favor and long for. To a healthy tongue, sugar candy is always sweet; unripe grapes taste sour. This we cannot change; if we do, it isn't the tongue that is doing the cheating! December is mighty cold on the icy slopes of Alaska; a den with a fireplace, however, is warm; night falls dark; sunrise illuminates; and the sea roars. All of these are furnished by our senses, just the way these things are.

One more special quality of the sense organs: our movements we can quantify and calibrate more or less accurately; not so, however, our sensations. They follow an "all-or-nothing" principle. A thunderbolt strikes our ears with intensity; whispers are faint; on a clear day, the high-noon sun is intensely bright;

in contrast, the later moonlight may be pale. All is faithfully transmitted without reduction or magnification, provided the transmitting organ is well. Any alterations are created by the gray matter of our brain.

Sense organs are purely receptive. Once their message is delivered, their job ends right there. Responses are not in their domain. Disregarding the continuous flow of information readily conveyed by our senses is tantamount to erasing moments, hours, days, perhaps years of our life. Misinterpreting their messages, we go astray. We may choose to see more, hear more, feel deeper. This is the noble function of all the arts, adding the dimensions of depth and breadth to the length of time traveled from birth to death. Time's confines thereby expand, accommodating more, with greater ease; an hour will last longer, be better.

Wherever our destiny or design takes us, form, sound, smell, taste and touch will meet us. With them we can make feathers fly and throats hum; we can make a hit or a miss; make little, make much; make peace or war; make believe or for real. We can soothe or bruise.

Every home comes with sunshine, moonlight, room, and a breeze; still, some homes seemingly dwell in darkness and are confining, with gloomy skies and mortifying air, their tenor unsettling and unusually heavy. Jo Hoshi (A.D. 382–414) summed it up: "All things are one's own making. He who realizes all things as himself is none other than a sage."[1] Don Juan, a Yaqui Indian seer from Sonora, Mexico told Carlos Castaneda, "The world is what we perceive, in any manner we may choose to perceive."[2] The choice is ours to make.

We may join hands with Andreyev in *The Life of Man*, where he condemns life so bitterly:

---

1. Quoted in Katsuki Sekida, *Zen Training* (New York: Weatherhill, 1981), p. 174.
2. Carlos Castaneda, *A Separate Reality* (New York: Pocket Books, 1972), p. 147.

I curse everything that you have given. I curse the whole of my life. I fling everything back at your cruel face, senseless Fate! Be accused, be forever accused! With my curses I conquer you. What else can you do to me? . . . With my last thought I will shout into your asinine ears: Be accused![3]

What a dreadful indictment of life! Or we may proceed with Thoreau: "I know that the enterprise is worthy. I know that things work well. I have heard no bad news." We can take either course. We may choose not to choose, and allow ourselves to be torn down by indecision, like Hamlet. In the early scenes, full of confidence, he announces: I know my course. Scenes later he vacillates, asking himself: Am I a coward? Finally he concedes: I lack ambition.

3. Quoted in D. T. Suzuki, *Essays in Zen Buddhism, First Series* (New York: Grove Press, 1978), p. 15.

Thought and Feeling: Are They Incompatible?
Are They Mutually Opposite?

THOUGHT OR FEELING? MUST WE CHOOSE? IF WE DO: at what price? Is it an *either-or* or an *and*? In the seventeenth century René Descartes, a brilliant mathematician, declared, *Cogito, ergo sum*: "I think, therefore I am." He believed that scientific knowledge was certain and that thought alone was the essence of human nature, adding that mind and body were separate entities, fundamentally different. Descartes' scientific certainty and analytic method of reasoning dominated Western culture and shaped the approach to science.

All but a century later, Jean-Jacques Rousseau shot back, *Sentio, ergo sum*: "I feel, therefore I am." Rousseau's celebrated writings and novels inspired the Romantic movement and had a profound effect on the leaders of the French Revolution. Aristotle's views, still held sacrosanct, promoted conflict and fostered opposition between thought and feeling, helped polarize their respective roles in human affairs and destiny. In his *Metaphysics*, Aristotle defended the principle of contradiction, condemning the doctrine of "All things are one" as absurd.

Hindu philosophers, Buddhists, and esoteric schools of Judaism, Christianity, and Islam didn't see things Aristotle's way. In the early nineteenth century, dialectics was resurrected and came to play a significant role in the West. Hegel, its noted champion, contradicted the principle of contradiction itself, viewing the Universe as a systematic whole rather than as an assemblage of mutilated fragments artificially separated from one another. He proposed *synthesis* for resolving conflict.

In the twentieth century the distinguished C. G. Jung challenged Sigmund Freud's view that conflict, hate, and fear drive humankind and dictate the course of civilization. Jung embraced both Western and Eastern philosophy and advised resolution of conflict and opposition through unity. Finally, physics of the twentieth century laid to rest the notion of absolute truth in science, proving that scientific theories are limited in scope and only approximate; instead, it called for a new approach toward the problems of reality.

Thought and feeling are not meant to replace or oppose one another. Thought stripped of feeling is austere, frosty, and dry. Feeling untempered by thought exposes our raw spots and makes us vulnerable to unforeseen events and uncontrollable circumstances. Complementing each other, thought and feeling are humanity's mark of distinction.

What propels the world and keeps it going is the interdependence of all opposites. Our own very survival depends on a delicate balance of opposites, counterpoised and working together in harmony. Every breath of life is a rhythmic inflation and deflation of our lungs. Every beat of our heart is a contraction and relaxation of our heart muscle. If contraction or relaxation stops, the heart will stop beating, blood circulation will come to a standstill, and death will follow within four or five minutes.

Bones and joints support our frame and ensure our mobility. Yet none of this can happen without the paradoxical action of so-called opposite groups of muscles: flexors/extensors; abductors/adductors; pronators/supinators; external rotators/ internal rotators; evertors/invertors. Muscular imbalance can create serious problems for us: inability to breathe, swallow, urinate, walk, write, drive a car, or open a door—to mention only a few. Our indispensable hormonal and enzymatic processes are merely a series of chemical reactions between activators and their respective deactivators. If they are altered ever so slightly, a host of grave illnesses will readily ravish us.

Consider inanimate objects: their elementary atoms and sub-atoms are in a state of perpetual motion; yet each object stays intact without fragmenting, and to our senses—in the absence of a propelling force—remains where it is. The equilibrium of forces cruising in opposite directions sustains the balance and visible stability of the Universe.

For many of us, the most troubling and most difficult thing

to comprehend or accept is the seeming interdependence of ''good'' and ''evil.''

> In the world, things are relatively ''good'' and ''evil,'' not absolutely so, since there can be no absolute qualities within creation. From another point of view, things are good and evil only in relation to us, not in relation to God, for in His eyes all things are performing but one task: making the Hidden Treasure manifest. Moreover, if there were no evil in the world, there would be no means whereby many of God's Attributes could manifest themselves, e.g., Forgiveness and Vengefulness. What sins could He forgive, and for what could He take vengeance. . . . God wills both good and evil but He only approves of the good. For God said, ''I was a Hidden Treasure, so I wanted to be known.'' Without doubt, God wills both to command and to prohibit.[1]

Religion is the product of unbelief. If there is no unbelief, why have religion? If the experience of evil does not occur in the first place, why try to avoid it? Indeed, how can we stay away from it, if it is nowhere in evidence? Not unrelated to these questions are God's perceived attributes of mercy, forgiveness, and their opposites—severity and punishment. With no sinners among us, there could be no saints, so that it is fair to say that the sinner makes the saint manifest, and the contrast furnished by the saint makes the sinner manifest. In this dualistic scheme of things, they need one another in order to appear at work in their respective roles. So when you burn a candle to the saint, don't forget to pray for the sinner!

The same goes for the healer and the infirm, the knowledgeable and the ignorant, the teacher and the pupil—one cannot perform without the other. Looking at things, our eyes are open, yet an invisible blinder frequently intervenes; thus we miss their true nature and the inherent coexistence of opposites

---

1. William C. Chittick, *The Sufi Path of Love: The Spiritual Teachings of Rumi* (Albany: State University of New York Press, 1983), pp. 53, 56.

everywhere. We become confused. Guided by the discriminating intellect, our intriguing mind keeps on classifying and dividing. Opposites are viewed as separate from one another, and opposition is perceived as a conflict to be resolved only through elimination of one or the other of the contending forces.

Inevitably all this leads to restlessness and continued strife—all-time human maladies. To its detriment and suffering, the human organism, by its own doing, is split into two contesting halves, and their continued friction ignites a fire from within—a fire that refuses to die. The wise transcend all opposites, for they see them performing their task, interdependent and not dissimilar.

With good and heedfulness alone, this world will fall to one side and collapse. It needs the bad and the heedless to stay in place the way we know it. Therein lies the spectrum of human compassion and equanimity. In embracing the opposites and accommodating the paradoxical, we rise above them rather than getting caught in between.

Descartes and Rousseau made far-reaching statements, yet in attempting to divide the indivisible, both notables missed the mark. *Truth is indivisible and therefore realizable only beyond the realm of opposites.* Only from this high point can the true nature of things and events be revealed. This is an essential component of Right Seeing.

Desire, Lust, and the Blues:
A Personal Experience

ALONE, STROLLING ON THE BEACH. PENSIVE, I STARTED
talking to myself. Here's what happened: casually I stopped by
a familiar rock, sat down, picked up a pretty seashell, and idly
watched the tide rolling in. Receptive, and dropping the customary guards that shelter oneself, the words of C. P. Cavafy,
the old poet of Alexandria, haunted me.

> There's no new land, my friend, no new sea,
> For the city will follow you: in the same
> Streets entangle endlessly, the same
> Mental suburbs slip from youth to age,
> In the same house go white at last—
> The city is a cage.
>
> No better landfall waits for you but this,
> No ship to take you—Ah! Can you not see
> How just as your whole life you've spoiled
> In this one spot, you've ruined its worth
> Everywhere now over the whole earth.[1]

As if this were not enough, Kali's song of sorrow started ringing in my ears like the hideous sound of a fitful alarm: "My
immaculate head has been fixed to the body of infamy, I desire
and do not desire, I suffer and yet I enjoy, I loathe living and
am afraid to die."[2] Caught in an invisible yet real and utterly
intriguing web from which escape is difficult, self-examination
seemed the right thing to do. I must have been ready for that.

1. Quoted in Lawrence Durrell, *Alexandria Quartet: Justine* (New York:
E. P. Dutton, 1961), p. 181.
2. From Marguerite Yourcenar, *Oriental Tales*, trans. Alberto Manguel
(New York: Farrar, Straus & Giroux, 1985), p. 124.

Without delay, an unseen door swung wide open, revealing the dreadful and the beautiful: violets, jasmine blossoms, black roses, cactus flowers, tumbleweed; hummingbirds; iguanas; big fish swallowing small fish; chickens running with their heads cut off; Hiroshima weeping, the Ota River sad, its seven branches flooding with charred bodies, ashes, and tears; man and the beast; man the beast; pairs of men and women stricken with desire, blazing lips, amateurish kisses, secret rendezvous, soft cooing propositions, naked torsos, moist armpits exhaling a complex aphrodisiac scent; cheap lipstick, dark eyes, ripening breasts longing to fall in the palm of a loving hand, sore tongues aching to meet in voiceless intimate dialogues; palpitations; throbbing genitals burning to conquer and surrender; thighs melting, hands trembling, arms like creeping vine on a rugged, hairy trunk; dancing silhouettes; fragmented vases; candles flickering out; infatuations, hurried ejaculations, broken promises; gold chains, diamond cufflinks, choking necklaces, fingers strangled by matrimonial rings; whores for sale, virgins desiring too ardently; inverted places, wasted times, intoxicating rituals; the Pacific plate moving north, the North American plate moving South, and the San Andreas fault shuddering in between, with only a wise crow and a distant kite knowing when a cataclysmic earthquake might erupt; wrathful, wounded Shahrayar spellbound by the magic of Shaharazad's unending Thousand and One Nights tale; Zeus, overcome by desire, disguised as a cuckoo and managing to ravish Hera, the disinclined queen of heaven; Lucifer rebelling from God; Sophia (wisdom) conceding her imperfection by yearning to unite with Him; and Adam and Eve bewildered and betrayed by knowledge.

This was in March. Venus passed Jupiter, and shortly after dusk I witnessed the planetary conjunction adorning the western sky, Venus bright and glittering, Jupiter imperial and aloof. Two hours after midnight, Saturn arrived, and thirty minutes later Mars followed, both gleaming, mysterious, and remote, all in the vicinity of the moon. Saturn stood between me and the center of the Milky Way, and almost by reflex I held my feet fast to the earth beneath lest I be lost to eternity.

Without a pause, I went right through the intertwine to where the eye of my mind was looking. There, I saw the downside and the downfall: anger, greed, jealousy, lust, and fear—all flashing red, signaling the abyss beyond. Instinctively I came to my own self-defense, pleading the mandate of necessity and the imperative of survival. To help prop myself up and recover esteem I began recalling attributes and deeds I have always considered good that perhaps would more than make up for the shortcomings. This maneuver failed to bail me out. Cavafy and Kali were still in charge. The two outwitted me.

There and then, I confessed to having given in to these blinding passions. In good conscience, with no further bickering or self-pity, I vowed to extinguish all, once and for all. Unyielding, the old Greek-Egyptian poet and the young Hindu goddess wouldn't budge nor clear the stage of my mind. The three of us must have been sharing something in common: affection, desire, transgression, imperfection—or it may just have been an incidental gravitational field that pulled us together. Whatever, for good or worse I was too weary to draw the curtain down. So the mental play went on, and for the remaining scenes, I continued my triple role as principal character, captive audience, and narrator of events.

Surrendering to compelling passions, my zestful arms reached out and my eager hands grasped and clung. Wouldn't let go. Desire bred desire and one contest hatched another, with no tranquility in sight. Winning, I immodestly rejoiced; losing, I came to grief. The euphoria of victory was sweet and brief, ending in itself, quickly swept away by dead-cold emptiness. With a vacuum to fill, apprehension and boredom slipped in like heavy, ominous clouds. Joys and sorrows propelled one another, up and down, back and forth like a seesaw. Caught in the treadmill, I continued running if only to keep the pace, but still no progress, no repose, no peace of mind. Always in square one, with more of the same, yet drained and dispirited.

Time after time I wondered if I was caught in the inevitable—if it was all a matter of fate. Could that be all there was to it? As I struggled to recover myself, and despite the row and the clamor, the remote sound of an old popular song filtered into the predisposed ear of my mind: "If that is all there is my friends, then let us keep dancing, break out the booze and have a ball." Listening in, the reanimated tunes furnished energy for peeling off layer after layer of memory. With so many tender fragments directly exposed, I began reexamining them to find their significant side. I seriously called into question the poignant lyrics: curing life's folly with dance and booze?!? Is that all I can do? Is that all there is? Ending folly with folly! Why bother? There must be a better way.

Am I a captive of space, time, and circumstance? A bird in a cage named existence? Is this what I am? My character, my will, my choice—are these real or illusion? Can I resolve the dilemma of being? Can I meet the obligatory challenges of survival and remain intact without compromising my very essence? Can the restless human soul find rest and peace on earth, or must it first travel to a realm beyond—where everyone seems to be heading—never to return, while we sit here speculating and hoping to hear from them? I must make up my mind: sink or swim, drift or navigate.

A whisper from without called in, faint, yet with the force of a powerful ultracentrifuge, so that it shook me to my marrow: "Did we come here to laugh or cry? Are we dying or being born?"[1] Within the same tidal wave, Blavatsky's *Voice of the Silence* thundered in: "Don't believe that lust can ever be killed out if gratified or satiated."

Physically still by the oceanside, glued to the same rock, my feet flirting with the cold water, my fingers and palms caressed the pretty shell. But my mind was far, far away, traveling its own journey at a speed faster than the speed of light. At the crossroads of infinity, seemingly on the threshold of the spaceless and the timeless, my own voice of silence recovered unusual tone and momentum. The internal dialogue picked up with force, drowning all external voices—rejuvenated, caring,

1. From Carlos Fuentes, *Terra Nostra* (New York: Penguin Books, 1978).

and kind. A new air of freshness came to town—the town within—and an awakening budged open a heavy rusty gate. Played back, here is what my voice of silence uttered:

Beware, living creature! Don't make your abode on shaky ground, for it cannot withstand the tempest and the deluge. Discard your easy pack of bandages and emollients. They won't heal self-inflicted wounds, gaping, draining, and deep. Tranquilizers, synthetic diversions, and trivial pursuits; what will they do for the tormented human soul? The hidden scroll of your true higher self, invisible for so long, is finally unveiled, flooded with a reading light that will never dim nor flicker, its original format preserved, legible. Read and remember! Don't let it go! In it nests your true capital, your pure essence. Material possessions, servants, maids, and chic company—all just a delusion and a trap. Fireworks with no real substance. In reaching out to help others is where true value resides.

Recovered soul: here is your agenda; read and remember it; fulfill some, fulfill all, fulfill *one*: work for healing the sick, sheltering the homeless, feeding the hungry, banning wars—all wars, clearing the human psyche of its morbid fascination with gunpowder and its suicidal obsession with nuclear bombs. Work for purifying the contaminated environment—air, rivers, oceans, soil, and whatever flows underground. Renew commitment to honoring and protecting life—all life, including that of your fellow-creatures, human and other. Foremost on your agenda: declare Truth and propagate the good word. Truth shall not be relative, shall not be conditioned by circumstance or tailored to our needs. We desperately need the original "undifferentiated" Truth before its distortion by human rationalization and double standards. *This is the path toward improvement of the human condition. End personal suffering and bring joy to the world!*

The Ego: Is It for Real? What Is It Doing in My Garden of Serenity?

WITH SO MUCH THAT HAS ALREADY BEEN WRITTEN and said about "ego," it is inconceivable to speak of *coping* without mention of what came to be the Latin for "I." And I begin by wondering whether this entity is real or false. Could it be a figment of the mind? Is it a spiritual substance of sorts grafted onto us way, way back, meeting no rejection—it "took" and became synonymous with self?

Looking inside ourselves courageously, without preconditions or hangups, how much of this intriguing private domain is ego (or ego-controlled) and how much is non-ego (or ego-free)? Is denial of the existence of an ego a possibly risky undertaking? And is it realistic or worthwhile? What does it take to do it? Personal courage? Knowledge? Proof—or blind faith? Heading in this direction, are we playing with fire? Could we get burned or perhaps lose our point of reference? Is it a weird prescription for self-annihilation? Question after question keeps bombarding the mind. To some, the proposition must be disturbing, or at the very least puzzling; to others, a much-ado-about-nothing. Let us consult the scholars.

A great many scholars have identified the ego as that portion of the human personality we experience as *self* or *I*. It is credited with perceiving, remembering, evaluating, planning, as well as responding to the external environment and society. Characteristically assertive, Sigmund Freud sliced the human mind into three territories: id, ego, and superego. Together they constitute the dynamics of the human mind. Be that as it may, a basic question remains: Is ego a demon from within? Or is it the old nonvanishing devil who for millennia has been marauding the Garden of Eden, seducing, misleading, and bringing shame and sorrow to the human race—a tireless (and tiresome) fellow traditionally held responsible for our mistakes, misfortunes, and shortcomings—? Does ego have any merit, goodness, beatitude? And can we do *with* it—or *without* it? Do we have any choice?

Buddhism emphatically denies the mere existence of an ego, declaring that it is nothing but an illusion (Maya). Buddhism unequivocally warns that ego is responsible for man's misconceptions about his own nature as well as that of others and the world. Orthodox religions in general speak of the ego in unflattering parables and metaphors, illustrating its sinister nature and cautioning the "egoist" what he is up against. C. G. Jung saw no harm in accepting the ego, provided it was integrated with the ego of others and the world. Among scholars and believers, ego acceptance or denial has provoked some of the most stimulating and significant debates. The pendulum keeps swinging, while the crowd remains on the sidelines, confused or merely uninterested.

Misinterpreted or rigidly espoused, either viewpoint can do harm on an individual or a global scale. Ego-rejection (or the non-ego principle), perceived as strict self-denial, may readily pass on to denial of others—a tragic failing, severing the noblest of all human bonds: compassion. Imagine what could happen as a result! Self-denial practiced with ardor and zeal can reach a saturation point of turning into a full-fledged obsession. Obsessed, we become fixed to our point of view, believing that we are performing great deeds. Caught in this fascinating pool of self-reflection, self-importance lures us into the path of worthless pursuits, our vital energy drained, with no significant return. In this cul de sac many hermits end up.

The Hui-neng Sutra[1] describes such a wasted state of affairs: "To seek enlightenment by separating from this world, is as absurd as to search for a rabbit's horn." Furthermore, Gautama Buddha himself counseled that for self-denial to be complete it has in itself to be also denied, otherwise it becomes a disease of the mind.

---

1. From *The Sutra of Hui-neng*, trans. Wong Mou-Lam (Boulder: Shambhala Publications, 1969), p. 34.

It appears to me that the vast majority of Westerners believe in the existence of an ego. Many revere it as a towering monument, indispensable for maintaining prestige, stimulating competition, and asserting one's individuality. This can land us in difficult straits. Why? From the beginning, the ego and the world are one. With the emergence of the human consciousness, our ego starts separating itself from the ego of others and the world. A false notion; yet many a notable thinker falls into this delusive crack.

I am not alone in this world. I recognize my own existence on becoming aware of yours. A philosopher once said, "I only know I have an opinion when you start arguing with me!" Everywhere, at all times, with and without good reason, people contend and dispute with one another. If they don't, they feel uptight or get bored. Is it their inner calling to prove themselves and be reassured of their own presence? The very debate itself confirms the falsehood of separate existence.

In astrology, the map of one's soul is the Universe. The wise person says: I came out of this world. The ignorant brags: I came into this world. The wise one, believing in the unity of all the ingredients, is compassionate, humble, admirably at ease with himself and others. The ignorant—wrathful, boastful, and callous, figuring himself to be on a mission to conquer and master—inflicts injury and pain on others, the world, and inevitably on himself, for he is part of what he is hitting at. The ignorant, deluded, repudiates the concept of life as One. Ever occupied in taking account of its innumerable manifestations, he fails to realize its ultimate oneness—the oneness of the many.

All being is interdependent. Alone, each is incomplete, incapable of independent survival. Life cannot be an exclusive entity. If it were so, who would then realize it? Life is a limitless whole, inclusive of all its components. Each component— every one of us included—is unequipped for independent survival. Who, therefore, can claim a separate reality? Only a fool would!

In the higher realms of true Suchness[2]
There is neither self nor other.
When direct identification is sought,
We can only say, Not two.
One in All,
All in One;
If only this is realized[3]
No more worry about you not being perfect.[4]

Rumi, a foremost Sufi scholar, put it succinctly this way: "You see two because you have gone astray and denied."[5]

2. Suchness is things as they really are in themselves without mental draperies and trappings.

3. Realization is frequently taken for understanding, but it is really personal experience through Right Seeing.

4. From *The Heart Sutra: Buddhist Wisdom Books*, trans. Edward Conze (London: George Allen and Unwin, 1980), p. 89.

5. William C. Chittick, *The Sufi Path of Love: The Spiritual Teachings of Rumi* (Albany: State University of New York Press, 1983), p. 84.

Sorrow and the
End of Sorrow

GAUTAMA BUDDHA, THE "AWAKENED," ONCE RE-
vealed to his disciples: "One thing I teach, O bhikkhus: sorrow and the end of sorrow." On attaining enlightenment, he
first chose not to pass it on to mankind; blinded by lust, humans would misinterpret his teachings. Finally, Brahma Shampoti himself pleaded with the Buddha not to enter upon Nirvana
at once without proclaiming the Dharma (Truth; doctrine).
"There are those," Shampoti argued, "who will understand."
The Buddha acquiesced, exclaiming: "The door is open to the
deathless." Out of compassion for humankind he deferred the
eternal bliss of Nirvana[1] and revolved the wheel of Dharma.

In the Four Noble Truths he pointed the way to end suffering: (1) the notion of individual, separate existence is inevitably bound up with *suffering*, or ill; (2) suffering has its
origination from *craving*; (3) there is a *stopping* of ill when craving has ceased; (4) the Eightfold Path leads to the cessation of
craving and therefore of ill. The long chain of suffering's cau-
sation he identified with one solitary link: ignorance. And it
is not ignorance in the sense of lack of conventional learning
or insufficient "head knowledge." This ignorance is *basal*. His
remedy for it is *Dharma*, Truth, which blooms in season and
out of season, evergreen, its branches rising high to the sun.

*First and foremost we must accept the world as it is: tran-
sient, constantly changing.* Its permanence as a whole, or for
that matter any part of it, is an illusion (Maya). Once this truth

---

1. Nirvana literally means "extinguishing," or cessation of ignorance and
limiting factors; its essence is awakening, revaluation, penetration, freedom
from growth and decay. Nirvana confers incomparable security. It is to be
found in the midst of this world.

concerning our world is realized, why cling to it? Why cling to anything? Clinging wastes our energy and inevitably leads to suffering. We cannot possibly secure everything we desire, yet desire and craving never seem to stop, and we are inclined to focus on what is "missing." Still, the verdict stands: all what we have and all what we have not, last not.

> Thus shall ye think of all this fleeting world:
> A star at dawn, a bubble in a stream;
> A flash of lightning in a summer cold.
> A flickering lamp, a phantom and a dream.[2]

Every path has its pitfalls. On this Path, one must be on guard not to cling to nonclinging! The right attitude is: neither indifference nor attachment to anything. One is thereby free without hindrance. Such is the essence of the principle of "non-attachment." It will set us free; we will function better and live better.

Next in order: *Our separate existence is falsehood, vastly contributing to our suffering.* We have already dealt with this, but it deserves restatement for emphasis.

Thirdly: *All teachings merely point to the goal but in themselves do not contain the goal.* Holy books and the sermons of prophets and sages do not, per se, hold wisdom. None of them *is* wisdom. They merely serve as pointers and clues. Wisdom and Truth cannot be packaged and delivered in words; they are inexpressible, realizable only through practice. A botany book may detail perfect descriptions of mangoes and apples, yet it does not supply a single mango or apple.

Followers and devotees who love to recite holy scriptures and who incessantly pray without practice are like a phantasm. Their toil is without cause, a classic case of self-deception. The surface may look sacred and perfect, yet the core reveals a most

---

2. From *The Diamond Sutra*, trans. A. F. Price (Boulder: Shambhala Publications, 1969), p. 74.

serious failing of religion and the religious. In their fervent zeal to affirm the faith, form and ritual are emphasized, pure essence is sacrificed, and the performance of good deeds is given a back seat.

Teachings are pure nonsense unless thoroughly understood, utterly useless unless personally realized and united to right action. It is strictly through one's own effort that wisdom and truth can be attained. This heraldic aspect of reality is alluded to by Jorge Luis Borges in *Dreamtigers*.

Then the revelation occurred: Marino saw the rose as Adam might have seen it in Paradise, and he thought that the rose was to be found in its own eternity and not in his words; and that we may mention or allude to a thing, but not express it; and that the tall, proud volumes casting a golden shadow in a corner were not—as his vanity had dreamed—a mirror of the world, but rather one thing more added to the world.[3]

Fourthly: *The principle of "Thusness" or "Suchness"* (Ta-thata) *implies realizing things as they are in themselves.* This is what they truly are—their Original Nature, so to speak—without the trappings and draperies cast by the mind that intrigues. Recognizing the opaque membrane veiling reality, the prophet Muhammad pleaded, "O Lord, show us things as they are!" By not going against the grain of things, we shall escape illusion and images, conserve energy, save time, and bypass disappointment and grief. Our path will become joyful. Because Thusness is the essence of mind.

Distracted by form, words, rituals, and metaphors, we fail to realize the true nature of religion. Each of these points a finger in a different direction, and we are misled. As a result, intolerance and blind hate plague our psyche, and from time to time savage wars erupt. Thomas Merton said, "All religions meet

3. Jorge Luis Borges, *Dreamtigers* (Austin: University of Texas Press, 1985, p. 38.

at the top." Jalal al-Din Rumi pointed out in the *Mathnewi*, "Every prophet and every saint has his own spiritual method, but it leads to God: All are one."

Gautama Buddha's prescription, briefly touched on in this chapter, serves as a sound model. Like a doctor's prescription, by itself it doesn't cure. *Application* is what counts. While Buddhism is not the only workable formula to end suffering, yet its study by non-Buddhists ought to help them understand and experience their own religions deeper and better. Many have found this to be true.

Ignorance and Knowledge

EXPANSIVE KNOWLEDGE OF BOOKS AND MANUSCRIPTS
—how valuable is it? How valid? Does it answer our questions
and fulfill our needs? Faced with life's challenges and never-
ending mystery, we pilgrim to lofty institutions of learning,
mind-setting libraries, and wizards of conventional knowledge.
We learn more and more about less and less, and our field of
vision narrows. Pursuing this path, we eventually become
specialists of one discipline or another, with blinders to right
and left. The rigmarole and turmoil of our existence never cease,
and with these thrown in, we almost cannot help but trip up.
On experiencing the fall, we habitually respond by spending
more time and effort along identical lines. This course of action merely brings more of the same without redress or satisfaction. Sincere seekers meet no contentment in this pursuit.

Relying exclusively on traditional knowledge and conventional understanding for guidance, we are not freely exercising the entire range of our potential. True, while plowing the
field of knowledge we are rewarded by spells of joy and fleeting glimpses of a world of fascination as we get to know what
we have not known before. Academic fever, scholastic laurels,
and diplomas on the wall intrude like creeping vines overpowering the oak tree.

To switch metaphors, in this euphoric state of mind the virus
of self-importance readily infects us, an opportunistic auto-
immune disease, insidious and subtle. As a result, our focus
of attention shifts to our self-image and we become our own
pampered child—an *enfant terrible*, indulgent and spoiled. Living in a bubble of inflated ego, we tread the surface of the earth
forward and backward flaunting our glorified image, inhaling
praise, exhaling arrogance and pride. Drawn to the circle of the
elite, we retreat behind high walls, advancing theories and inventing elaborate concepts to reorganize the universe. Full of

ourselves, we repeat in pride, "Behold, I know," rather than humbly confessing: "Thus have I heard."[1] I'm sure I have done some of this shameful bragging myself! But now, as the character in John Osborne's *Martin* exclaims, "I'd rather be able to see." I'd rather experience life as it is—its mystery, its grandeur, its chaos, charade, harmony, absurdity, and transiency. At this moment the big question cries out loud, begging for an answer: Are time, place and circumstance our undisputed masters, our unavoidable adversaries? Or are they our allies and helpers?

The bell long stilled in my heart starts swinging and ringing, summoning me to homecoming. Reared in the halls of conventional knowledge, time after time I have turned a deaf ear to this genuine sound. But this time I won't. I'll go searching for the rest of me, the real me, too long driven into hibernation by the blizzards of the mundane and the overpowering forces of the conventional. Self-examination, and not self-recrimination or fixation, is the way to self-knowledge, the real key to the fundamental truth about ourselves, others, and the world. The engine that takes us around must be studied, understood, and maintained in good working condition. This is what self-knowledge is all about.

The homecoming journey is not for the frivolous or the meek; it is a warrior's path. Still, we all have what it takes. It does not signal introversion and withdrawal. On the contrary, it is a self-liberating expedition. In parting with habit and routine, we are initially bound to be shaky, likely to feel ill at ease and a bit lonely as well. Foreseeing hardship and toil, shall we go ahead—or retreat and continue losing ourselves to a wasteland of oblivion? Shall we set out on the first stage of this long journey—or remain adrift at the mercy of circumstance, sailing the high seas of existential darkness, where sorrow knows no end? We are at a place of decision. Each must choose his, her, own way.

1. "Thus have I heard" is the formula traditionally used at the beginning of Buddhist scriptures.

On the March: Look What They Have Done to the Children— An Eyewitness Account

ON THE ROAD, THEN, LET US BOW TO THE CHILDREN of the world. Virgin is their sky, their air, innocent and placid, their colors raw and bright. Among them rows and squabbles do arise; they can wrangle and scuffle with one another. Nevertheless, left alone, their contentions readily melt away, and back they are again with one another, joyous and free. As they grow up, we begin to mold them our way, and the mantle of conformity is thrown over their eyes. Our social values, traditions, and stiff system of education beleaguer them, hardening the pliable and taunting the beautiful.

We continue on our mental march. There, where the river bends, a school complex looms on the horizon, pale in the distance. Shall we go, see for ourselves? Actually, the show is but a rerun of what most of us were put through. Scores of children are now being stacked for the authoritative programming of their minds. In the hushed classroom, school curricula are doled out, with little regard to aptitude or appetite. And if they don't like it, they must lump it. Slowly but surely their receptive, congenial mind turns into a hustle-and-bustle brimful of chemistry, geometry, mathematical equations, symbols representing other things, metaphors transferring to one word the meaning of another, opposites constantly refuting one another, paradoxes made irreconcilable (never to harmonize, never to embrace), definitions determining the limits, meaning, and properties of all things.

Spontaneous self-expression is done away with; there is no more telling it like it is, no more revealing one's genuine thought and true feeling. The process and way of telling become more consequential than what is to be told. Words must

42

be carefully picked, rehearsed, and coated with sugar. Responses must be precisely measured, skillfully targeted with synthetic courtesy. Most of all, real intentions must be disguised.

The children's heads in paper bags, the history teacher now enters. His or her personal preferences, racial bigotry, national zeal, and religious prejudice are all blended in with the story. Magnificent events are resketched, dwarfed, or deleted altogether; sequences are shuffled and reshuffled, motives of opportunity instilled, and the original script is tailored to fit the design. Real heroes and heroines are eclipsed; instead, villains and clowns are awarded the trophy, given the pedestal and crown.

Conquerors and organizers of mass slaughters are idolized, called "liberators," their ghastly crimes seemingly divinely inspired. Race always figures high on the agenda, the superiority of one's own race fostered and legitimized. The exclusive righteousness of a particular creed is emphasized and flag-worship sanctified. The burning flames of patriotism are fanned with glowing ballads, fiery anthems, and music. The national map is to be engraved on the citizen's heart, never to shrink, ever amenable to expansion dictated by imagined national interest, national security, or the leader's whims and dreams. Motherland, sweet motherland—passionate, restless, distressingly thirsty, ever lusting for the warm blood of her young. Red blood alone, it would seem, can quench her thirst, recover her dignity, and heal her pride.

Ladies and gentlemen: look at what they have done to the children! Their world of peace, love, mirth, and intuition turns into hell, with the brutal beasts of suspicion, fear, and strife obliterating the light and ravaging the garden and meadow.

Innocence and Knowledge: Are They Incompatible? Can We Have Both?

TIME, NOW, TO CONTEMPLATE THE HAPPY AND THE sad. In quiet recollection, memory opens up, effortlessly displaying the whole play for the eye of the mind to review and reconsider. One thing you notice is that childhood merriment, spontaneous and sweet, is now past. See how heavy and burdened the buoyant children have become. Their ingenious receptors are now plugged up, their bright colors are shifting to gray. Wholehearted laughter has gone flat, innocent, easy smiles have transformed into nervous reserve, and nature's music has fallen silent. Evil has truly been served, all the while history's verdict endures in the words of W. H. Auden: "Those to whom evil is done do evil in return."

Generation after generation humankind has been sentenced by this harsh verdict. Witness the long, unending trail of sorrow and tears. Millennium after millennium; no reprieve, always more of the same. And we never cease to wonder: is there no end to it? The path has been unhappy, always retracing itself. Caught between the most ominous mirrors, human action pathetically copies the past. Hope remains eternal, despair is neither fair nor justified; and there must be a way out of this ghastly hall of mirrors. But where shall we start? Where can the great work begin? Attempting to change adults' modes of thinking and behavior is onerous, perhaps even impossible. Tried and tried again, it seems never to have worked out.

If noble change is to be actualized, we must begin at the very beginning, right where the mischief first began. We must go back to the uncontaminated world of children—before they inherit the rule of the world. First, then, let us return their childhood, give them back what we have robbed them of, repair their injury before the scars of their psyche and the defor-

44

mities of their intellect become permanent. A mission momentous yet indispensable if humanity's pursuit of happiness is to materialize.

At the outset, certain formidable questions stand out. What went wrong? Is learning ("head knowledge") the culprit? Does it stand to be accused alone, or are there other transgressors? What is this knowledge? Is it the "Forbidden Fruit"? Did humankind trade innocence for knowledge, precipitating the "Fall" from grace, the exile from paradise? If so, whose fault is it? Who is responsible? Did Eve do Adam in? Did Adam vacillate or conspire? Were they both taken in and tricked by a mischievous third party? Are they sinners? Victims? Sinners *and* victims?

What about their children? Guilty to begin with—or innocent if and until they do wrong? Does it help or hinder to start life with a guilty conscience? Is the mark of Cain a universal condemnation or a note of caution to us all? The snake, the apple, the devil, and knowledge—do they leave a common trail? Are they feeding on each other? Are they one and the same? Did it all really happen the way we are told, or is it all parabolic and metaphorical? Does it matter? Since anything could have happened or might still happen, it is the significance of the happening that really counts. For that, to argue articles of faith is foolhardy.

"Head knowledge," the traditional form of knowledge, with which we all become familiar, is gathered in a linear manner, piecemeal. While acquiring it, human intelligence unintentionally transforms into something like a linear scanner, not too different from a computer. This goes on at the conscious level, while the brain as a whole continues to function as an integrated unit. It constantly receives, deals with, and assimilates a continuous flow of events and information, some of it freighted with great complexity and many variables.

A great wealth of information piles up, whether we want it to or not. This colossal treasury, possessed by everyone, is not subject to recall by our ordinary conscious mechanism. Our means of deducting, recombining, and recalling bits and pieces —acquired through learning—fail to unlock the safe. The story of the king of Benares and the blind beggars dramatizes the ineffectiveness of this approach. For lack of a better illustration, I use this almost worn-out tale, with apologies to those who have read or heard the story time and again.

Bored and despondent, the king summoned to his palace a number of beggars blind from birth. He offered substantial rewards to the beggar who might give the best description of an elephant. One beggar touched the elephant's leg and noted that the elephant was like the trunk of a tree. A second beggar, laying hold of the tail, announced that an elephant was like a rope. A third established contact with an ear and reported that the elephant was like a palm leaf. One beggar after another described the elephant by that part with which he came in contact. The blind beggars ended by disputing and quarreling with one another. Needless to say, the king was diverted and amused.

This story bears a certain resemblance to our educational system and to our conventional approach to knowledge. It comes, then, as no surprise that our education takes so long and accomplishes so little, the graduates a flock of flamingoes standing on one leg with vanity mirrors, face masks, and wearing colored goggles. Unable to see things as they are, yet all the while unwitting, they talk, talk, talk—and say nothing. Beholding others who see things differently, they act surprised and wonder why. Their response is either one of apathy, scornful silence, or a twist of mock modesty. Contempt, malicious laughter, and other signs of the siege mentality surface. Bitterness and hostility often follow.

Reconstructing the whole by adding its constituent parts together doesn't always work. More often than not, the result is "a horse of a different color." Dog-paddling or actually swimming in the vast sea of knowledge, we learn what we encounter, all subject to our approach and state of mind. Generally, we do not have a choice. Schooling, curricula, ways of teaching and learning are all mandated by society. The system is built on dissecting any one thing into minute fragments called units or subjects. The student is taught each fragment separately, the mind focusing on what is offered. In the process, the picture *as a whole* slowly fades away, dims, is eventually obliterated and forgotten. We who went through the rigmarole are left grabbing pretty fragments and broken pieces.

In effect, we become the king's blind beggars. Each of us with eyes wide open on coming in contact with a part of the elephant (knowledge) proudly thunders out, "I have it! I got it! It's such and such." A tree trunk; a rope; a palm leaf. Pieces. Parts. Fragments. That is all! Imagine gluing the tree trunk, the rope, and the palm leaf together with someone pointing: *There is the elephant of Benares!*

Preposterous and ludicrous as this is, it exemplifies our conventional approach to reality. No wonder we disagree so often, quarrel, and commit major errors one after another. Apologetically we murmur to ourselves: We can't help it . . . that is the way it is . . . we turn around and do it again.

Reality's innumerable components cannot be grasped or comprehended through linear or segmental thinking. Seers see *the whole picture.* Automatically the parts unfold like the petals of a flower, revealing themselves to discerning eyes. Fascinating (always mind-boggling to the rest of us how much seers seem to know), the stream of their knowledge appears endless. Indeed it is. They have reached the Source. "Coming home," they know themselves, they know the Universe as well; a bridge has been established with the macrocosm, the microcosm also freely communicating, unified with the Source. Staying open all the time, their mind never jams.

What we suspect to be intuition, hunch, premonition, they consider "The Doctrine of the Heart," "True Knowledge," "Soul Wisdom," facts of life. They read the past, see the present, and predict the future. It is all a continuum on which they look, in which they wander, and over which they preside. With amazing precision they foresee the moment of their death, advise their disciples of future events, and entrust the essence of their teaching to the select among them. Of course, the blind adherents, and literal-minded scholars are distracted by the mere words and engulfed in rituals.

What I am calling Source is never denied the sincere seeker. The door to True Knowledge ("Soul Wisdom") is open to the wayfarer who takes heart. "This is no journey for the feet, however. Look into yourself, withdraw into yourself and look," said Plotinus. The way most of us live, it is only natural that we function far below our capacity and expectation, yet remain restless, tired, and bored. Norman Cousins, a contemporary seer, concludes that human capacity is what it has to be. Limitations are human-made and for the most part self-imposed.

Seers of the past were obviously eyeing the same thing— Reality. Regardless of its many forms, irrespective of time and place, its essence is always One. The ignorant, caught and deluded by form, are derailed, fail to reach the core, and thus overlook the meaning. In the seventh century A.D., Hui-neng, the sixth patriarch of Zen, wrote, "The capacity of the mind is as great as that of space—it is infinite." His teachings and doings only confirm the validity of his statement.

The only way out of our quandary is by freeing the will. Don Juan identified the will as "a force which is the true link between men and the world." He further added: "Will is a power within ourselves. It is not a thought, or an object, or a wish. . . . Will is what can make you succeed when your thoughts tell you that you're defeated. Will is what makes you invulnerable. Will is what sends a sorcerer through a wall; through space; to the moon, if he wants."[1] And Hui-neng says: "If you turn your light inwardly, you will find what is esoteric *within you.*"[2]

With will and mind united, we will experience the mystery and grandeur of life, and our abilities will know no limits.

1. Carlos Castaneda, *A Separate Reality* (New York: Pocket Books, 1972), p. 147.
2. From *The Sutra of Hui-neng*, trans. Wong Mou-Lam (Boulder: Shambhala Publications, 1969), p. 21.

Realizing the true spiritual essence of our nature, the unrealized immense human potential will come into being, and the hidden seer in every one of us will emerge. Our heroes and heroines, poets and prophets, wizards and outstanding scientists—all the gifted ones—are but you and I without fear, self-doubt, or self-imposed restraints. For all these are brought about by ignorance—ignorance of our very self. And ignorant, we stray, we stumble, we lose.

The work of the Ear ends with Hearing,
The work of the Mind ends with Ideas.
But the Spirit is an emptiness ready to take in all things.

—Chuang-tzu

Lost and Found

WANTING AND WISHING ALONE WON'T DO IT FOR US. *It must be willed*. Everybody wishes to be happy, healthy, handsome, beautiful, and wise. Yet only the few *will* their wishes. Still, each of us has his or her own resources, with no one having the authority to dictate to us which way to go. The fact is: *we all have the ingredients to make it*. Dig them out. The pearls lie inside, and the bottom line is doing what we realize to be true.

We should not put off this most important undertaking to a later time. Procrastination and hesitation kill momentum. Let us rearrange ourselves right now. No doubt we can do much better for ourselves and for others. We must forget what *has* happened, no more worrying about what *will* happen, and take what *is* happening. Everyone—everyone—can lay some happiness on the world. Everyone can light the lights. Fly an attitude of expectancy. Begin now.

Time is fleeting, learning is vast; no one knoweth the duration of one's life.[1]

1. W. Y. Evans-Wentz, ed., *Tibetan Yoga and Secret Doctrines* (London: Oxford University Press, 1935), p. 62.

PART TWO
ON BEING CREATIVE AND FREE

The Path is beautiful and joyful and familiar.

—Meister Eckhart

To be free from the illusion that we are not free . . .

—R. H. Blyth

But that there is really nothing to disturb my serenity . . .

—Shou-an

To Be Free

TO BE FREE IS TO LIVE LIKE THE ROSE, WHICH, ACCORD-
ing to Meister Eckhart, lives without a why. To be free is to
eat when you are hungry, rest when you are tired, slumber when
drowsy, go when you decide to go, or come and stay on as you
wish. To be free is to plan your plan, choose your choice, and
follow your path. To be free is to break away from the bondage
of fear, the torment of anxiety, the unfairness of bias, the
uncertainty of ambiguity, the burden of hate, the snare of lust
and the self-destruction of stress.

To be free is to drop down the mask that has disguised your
original face for so long. To be free and creative is to recognize
your original face and let your true, benevolent nature manifest
and shine. To be free is to live by the prescription of R. H. Blyth,
"To think only and entirely and completely of what you are
doing at the moment, and you are free as a bird." All the while
performing your task effectively, genuinely caring, and joyfully
inclined—whether residing in a sprawling metropolis, an exclusive suburb, or a remote, forlorn town.

> Nothing is there to come, and nothing past,
> But an eternal now does everlast.
>
> —Abraham Cowley

To realize a state of this kind we must integrate mind and
body under the auspices of our free will. This is no empty talk
to stuff the hollow and cheer the pessimist. It is no abstrac-
tion, either. All is real, practical and within reach, even though

it may seem like a fanciful vision of a daydream, too good to be true.

It is a great joy to realize that the path to freedom which all Buddhas have trodden is ever existent, ever unchanged, and ever open to those who are prepared to enter upon it.

—Precepts of the Gurus[1]

Together let us experience the joy and mystery, the mystery and joy of living, which in the eye of human folly is seen as a phantom and a reverie.

---

1. *The Diamond Sutra*, trans. A. F. Price (Boulder: Shambhala Publications, 1969), p. 11.

The Meadows Are Calling:
The Story of Humankind's Longest March

IT IS SPRINGTIME, THE DAY IS SOFT, THE MORNING
air is mild, the meadows are calling—green and pleasant, inviting us for a stroll. Trees are in flower and the sun is breaking through the clouds. After the benediction of the rain, the
air is fresh, crisp, and clear, and I can see the impression of
my foot on the soil softened and pampered by the rain. As I
look closer and closer at the earth beneath, I clearly recognize
my footprint: the mark of my heel, the outline of my foot arch,
and the contour of my abducted big toe. All characteristically
human. In the morning peace, man's erect posture and the long
trail of his footsteps, stretching unbroken, regale my eyes. With
these comes the memory of man's grandeur and folly; his endearing tenderness and compassion; his cruel betrayal of his
covenant with life, fellow-humans and other creatures; his august memory; his pathetic forgetfullness of his humble begin-
nings; his passionate ties to family, land, and river; his mindless
severing of ancestral roots deeply embedded in gene, rock, and
soil.

Right in the midst of these paradoxes, a flashing light sig-
naled all of a sudden. Following the light, as though by reflex,
my mind headed east. Afar, in the mystical wastelands of
Egypt's Sahara, my mind's eye caught a glimpse of the "dawn
ape"—the enigmatic, arborial Aegyptopithecus roaming the
lush tropical rainforest of the historical Faiyum Depression,
now barren and desolate. At the breathtaking distance of 33
million years, I could clearly see the perplexed creature staring me in the face, the enclosed eye sockets unmistakably
human-like, and with 32 teeth added to the fascinating riddle.
This energetic nine-pound ape, which subsisted on nuts and
fruits, is now considered the direct ancestor of man by emi-
nent scholars such as Dr. Elwyn Simons of Duke University.

Treading man's route in reverse, the road was long, trails were elusive and treacherous, mountains high and stubborn, forests thick and forbidding, sand quick, the still mud quietly swallowing the timid and the brave. The deep, gutsy rivers rushed swiftly, and the carnivorous beast kept on cracking the bones and feasting on the flesh. Hailstones came with violent hurricanes, and dark, heavy rain ushered in the flood, with mosquitoes, pestilence, and famine giving agony its story to tell. The wheel of time perpetually turns, patiently unfolding and shaping the destiny of man.

Six to seven million years ago a momentous event took place: the "Terminal Myocene Event"—a profound chill devastated the continent of Africa and permanently split apart hominid and his ancestor pongid. Man was now forced to abandon arborial existence for a terrestrial one. He had to go it alone. Quitting the ape's side-to-side loping and its bent-knee gait, he finally walked erect, with head upright. Fossil fragments from Kenya, Tanzania, and Ethiopia tested by a radiometer that measures the rate of potassium decay into argon unveiled impressive details.

Wondrous encounters are, for the most part, the work of chance, arising in the pursuit of other things. Contrariwise, the path of the serious scholar is long and wearisome, but ultimately fulfilling in many ways. A certain day in November 1976 was, for anthropologist Donald C. Johnson, a most intriguing, most influential date. It all concerned a young lady from Hadar in Ethiopia. At the early age of 25, her tender body was laid to rest in an unmarked grave. Over millennia her bones remained, destined to make a statement, far-reaching and profound. Withstanding the wear and tear of 3 million years, the lady's dainty skeleton held on to its distinctive form and unique texture—furrows, ridges, bony canals, foramina all remarkably preserved. In her, experts recognized a new species: Australopithecus afarensis.

Not to forget the young lady herself, the scholarly group named her Lucy after the then-popular Beatles song "Lucy in the Sky with Diamonds," a witty gesture linking science and

56

the pop arts. The famous Taung child unearthed 50 years earlier in a South African mine was subsequently put in the same species with Lucy. Born 1 to 2 million years after her, the well-known African child made it only to a very young age, five or six. His skull survives to this day, in eloquent silence overlooking both time and space and telling a substantial part of the story of humankind.

Modern men and women pay homage to Africa, our motherland for being the undisputed birthplace of the human race. Anguished and oppressed, the "dark continent" is frequently abused and despised by its "civilized" sons. But we should make no mistake: there, in the primordial African cradle, and nowhere else, we evolved and were made to survive the ravages and havoc of our environment. For millions of years the tormented continent was the sole home on planet earth known to our predecessors, the four species of Australopithecus—afarensis, africanus, robustus, and boisi—and to Homo habilis and Homo sapiens as well.

Homo erectus evolved 1.6 million years ago. With a body stature closely approximating our present size, a brain averaging 1000 grams (milliliters, to be more precise), and an assortment of specialized stone tools, erectus dared to wander further than the end of Africa. His perseverance and upright march took him to the remote lands of China, Indonesia, and Southern Europe. Homo sapiens succeeded him. In possession of a larger brain (1350 ml.) and better tools, he kept on walking, bravely making his way to Northern Europe and chilly Siberia, later crossing the Bering Strait to North America 30,000 to 50,000 years ago—all without driving chariots, mounting horses, or riding camelback. Only recently in Syria and Egypt did man domesticate animals (8000 B.C.) and invent the wheel (3500 B.C.).

Why Bother with Lucy, the Taung Child, and a Number of Toys Called African Fossils?

AT FIRST SIGHT, BRINGING UP A WEIGHTY SUBJECT such as the origin of man, his roots, and wanderings—spanning millions of years—appears excessive. Yet it occurs to me that the awe surrounding it might lend credit and perhaps a touch of splendor to an otherwise mundane subject. From the very first to the present, and from here to all eternity, the human spirit is a continuum, unbroken. The remote shadows of our forebears recruited for the script might kindle in us a sense of belonging; a forgotten affinity for mother earth; love for trees and forests; comfort in rivers and streams; blessedness in rain and early-morning dew upon cold sleepy flowers; respect for Africa, her people, and the dispossessed tribes of our era; a passion for walking again, dancing, exercising, moving about and tuning into nature's wavelength and the rhythm of time.

The determined footprints of our ancestors adorned the surface of all five continents. The uninhabitable thick forests, the forbidding badlands, the impassable mountain ranges did not halt their march. Pity, we, their modern-day offshoots (more or less), have forgotten how to move about. The more so in the industrialized nations: people are growing notoriously harder and stiffer, knees getting callous, spines becoming hunched and rigid, bellies softer and bigger, hips complaining and crackling under the merest strain. The slightest imbalance hurls us to the ground, fracturing our brittle bones and snapping our atrophied ligaments.

Blindly and recklessly we have pawned our marvelous locomotor system, with the vast freedom it affords, for a naive dependency on locomotor engines. The 4-million-year glory of bipedalism has been foolishly surrendered to the idleness of cars, buses, trains, and lifts. The thought of climbing up a hill or mounting the staircase is a bother and a bore. What a drag!

Uncalled-for! Leisurely trotting down a slope—why bother? A stroll in a park or an early-morning walk by the oceanside? You gotta be kidding! "My feet hurt! These shoes are killing me!"

Locked indoors together with our electronic gear, we sink into the comfort of lazy-boy chairs glued to witless television sets and dumb video screens. The penalty is imperative and compelling, and serves us right. Unused calories turn to fat. As we tend to obesity, diseases and disabilities of all kinds afflict us: arthritis of the hips, knees, and spine; diabetes mellitus; cancer of the breast, uterus, colon, and pancreas; high blood pressure and heart attacks. Society as a whole pays dearly.

Deserted streets, lonely sidewalks, vacant playgrounds, abandoned public parks disintegrate into pastures for thugs and muggers—a no-man's-land where one ventures at one's risk. The environment is victimized too, with the automobile heading the sinister long list, the number-one air polluter. Our lungs and hearts grow tired and indisposed as our big cities lie pitifully suffocating beneath thick blankets of smog that veil the blue sky, bleach the rainbow, obliterate the horizon, and eclipse the sun. We are not using our automobiles; they are using us.

The same could be said for radios, television sets, tape players, and VCRs. Are we still masters of these wonderful machines? What can one say? We scarcely talk to one another because we rarely stroll together. Television and radio are doing the talking for us. Tapes are "rapping." Technology is replacing memory. Diminished to a pack of lonely strangers, we become unknown to others—and to ourselves as well. Our hurried pace leaves no room for calmness, thoughtful deliberation, or joyful recollection. We have established the perfect setting for tension and stress, the deadliest and most prevalent malady of our time.

> . . . the race is not always to the swift;
> . . . there is more to life
> Than increasing its speed.
>
> —Orin L. Crane

Walk Softly: The Ethics and Artistry of Walking—A Point of View

STROLLING ALONG, LET OUR FOOTSTEPS FALL SOFT and light. Grace and good manners are sufficient reasons; but— perhaps with some acquiescence on your part—let our reason be one of *reverence*. Reverence for our forebears and for all the other creatures of times gone by. Their mortal frames rest in the entrails of mother earth together with fallen leaves, worms, rocks, and suchlike things. With humility and elegance, Al Maarri, the great Syrian poet and mystic, tenderly unveiled these subtleties in memorable works, including *The Tinder Spark*; *The Necessity for the Unnecessary*; and *Risalat-Al Ghufran*. By a stroke of good fortune, G. Brockenbury translated the *Risalat* in 1943; later it became known to the West as *A Divine Comedy*—an engaging treat for the English reader seeking literature of substance and high taste. The poet narrates his personal experience as he journeys through hell and paradise, becoming acquainted with his predecessors, who were forgiven their past sins. From his works certain verses on the artistry and ''ethics'' of walking fairly beg to be told.

O pigeon perching on a tree branch melodiously swinging
with the wind:
Weeping, are you? Singing? I wonder!
Friends, come to; bear witness:
Our graves have pressed the far-reaching lands.
These whereabouts are graves from times long gone by.
Step lightly, will you! Our mortal bodies make the crust
of the earth.
Fellows and chums, doubt not.

Shame and pain if we continue desecrating our fathers
and forefathers.
Softly ride the wind, surrender your haughty, awkward steps.[1]

Al Maarri was blinded in early childhood, yet his vision reached farther and penetrated deeper to planes invisible than it does with those blessed with the gift of sight. Like a spider in seclusion, this immortal seer toiled in solitude, spinning poems steeped in wisdom, radiating beauty and charm, their verses affectionately reaching us across a time barrier of more than 900 years.

Three centuries later, Dante Alighieri wrote *The Divine Comedy*—an account of his voyage through Hell guided by Virgil, then into Purgatory, and on to Paradise with Beatrice, his spiritual love. Somewhere, somehow, perhaps more likely than not: on his sojourn Dante met his immortal predecessor Al Maarri. Of this we are not told. Both poets walked the same path. And we inherit the verses.

1. Author's rendering.

Feet and the Soil

RIGHT THIS MINUTE IF YOU FEEL LIKE WALKING, GO ahead. Listen to your feelings, obey your own call. Go on. And turn the excursion into a graceful act. On a trail joyfully trod in childhood; by a secluded lakeshore where once you met a friend; along the familiar banks of your native river; down the "mean streets" of your city childhood; upon a new hill or in the forgotten greenfield of a countryside—spring or fall, summer or winter, night or day: move on, free, with no restraints. Let your hangups and your worries wait. Better still, leave them behind. Concentrate; focus your mind on the present moment and what you are doing now.

Let your walking feet feel the very soil they are now treading over; get acquainted with the earth; experience its yielding texture, many cracks, uneven contours, moist grass, velvety moss, cool damp surface at dawn, pebbles, loose gritty sand, hard rocks and the like. At such a time your feet become your feelers, private antennas of a kind. Their dainty muscles are numerous, busy contracting and relaxing, with each single muscle fiber always contracting to its maximum. These muscles deserve special recognition, and much good will come of such recognition.

Don't neglect your muscles; don't slight them! In matters of survival, they have a big say. This may sound like an exaggerated claim, but in truth, it isn't. The heart—tender, warm, and loving—is but a diamond-shaped muscle. The diaphragm, which draws the breath of life in and out—what is it? A thin, expansive sheet of muscle. Muscles allow us to swallow, urinate, defecate, talk, sing, and smile.

In what follows I shall try to elaborate, bringing to light what our muscles can offer to improve performance and maintain well-being. They are more than plain, dumb contractile elements—much more. From now on, let's relate to them and regard them with respect.

62

Our Survival and
Our Internal Environment

WE LIVE IN TWO ENVIRONMENTS—ONE EXTERNAL, the other internal. For survival, the external environment must be *endurable*, the internal *even* and *constant*. The external environment exists outside the confines of our integument— limitless, changeable, and with many elements: air, water, fire, earth, plants, galaxies, animals, people, and many more.

The internal environment is our private domain, a sheltered citadel beneath our skin and mucous membranes. There, decisive action takes place where the omnipotent Vital Force works its miracles, giving us life, warmth, feelings, intellect, and that which makes us human. And there we find an awesome assembly of juices, ferments, body fluids, warm blood, emotions, passions, desires, sexual drive, breath cycles, fairly constant body temperature, heartbeat, hormonal balance, specific biochemical states; in short, what have you. Our internal atmosphere is very well conditioned and finely attuned to the most trivial interventions. The slightest misadjustment manifests itself in one serious infirmity or another, unrelenting pain, or even the cessation of life itself.

A highly specialized area of the brain known as the limbic system is entrusted with the indispensable task of keeping our internal environment constant. As a matter of necessity, this system is highly developed in all mammals. Its most influential member is the hypothalamus, a pearl located in the center of the brain. Performing multiple intricate functions, it weighs a mere four grams. Since it plays a crucial role in keeping us conscious and awake, besides having thought-controlling powers, the hypothalamus is very important to our discussion. Its many other functions are beyond the scope of this book.

Our Wandering Thoughts:
Can We Control Them?

WHILE AWAKE, WE EXPERIENCE WAVE AFTER WAVE of wandering thoughts. They never seem to stop. To stay calm or in order to concentrate, we try and try to chase them away. The harder we try, the less successful we are in bringing these tiny intruders into line. Somehow they manage to sneak in, bypassing our defenses. As a result, the mind, though longing for harmony and peace, remains restless, at odds with its own product thought. This predicament is not new; it began way back. With the progressive evolution of the brain, second, third, fourth, and many more thoughts were born—a dramatic development forcing us into making choices and paying attention. Life became more complex, and the problem is now one of abundance.

The logical solution would appear to be thought-control; regulation, if you will, by the individual himself, not by society or the state. With no magic on-and-off switch, the challenge seems substantial. I see the hypothalamus as the key. In 1837, Hawthorne wrote to Longfellow: "I have made a captive of myself, and put me into a dungeon, and now I cannot find the key to let myself out." Quoting Lawrence Durrell, "I know that the key I am trying to turn is in myself."

Controlling Our Thought: A Key Factor in Conquering Stress with Recovery of Freedom and Creativity—The Available Mechanism

THE HIGHER BRAIN CENTERS IN CHARGE OF THE thinking process by themselves dismally fail to regulate or control thought. To accomplish this most important undertaking, the hypothalamus and body muscles must be brought into play, fulfilling their supportive and interdependent roles. A highly developed two-way traffic system brings the two to function as an integrated unit. Mixing my metaphors, I may say that the fulcrum and keystone of this sophisticated network is the hypothalamus. Both the higher brain centers and muscles can stimulate the hypothalamus; in return, the hypothalamus is capable of stimulating both.

Physical effort—be it walking, running, swimming, dancing, or even simple deep breathing—generates a certain degree of tension in participating muscles. Muscular tension is transformed into electric signals that travel the special pathway to the hypothalamus. On arrival, they initiate a state of heightened awareness with thought-controlling capability. On this account, the hypothalamus earned a distinctive title: *the wakefulness center*. Our mind concedes that thought unaided cannot control thought, and whenever it wishes to govern its own thought, it calls on our muscles for help.

A simple experiment requiring no equipment confirms the inability of the mind alone to check thought. In a secluded place sit down with the intention of not thinking anything whatsoever. Almost as soon as you begin, an idea or thought of one sort or another will rush to your mind, throwing off your attention. Realizing what has happened, you will try again to stop thinking. In a matter of seconds another idea will come along, engaging you. As you continue the experiment, you will repeat this pattern over and over, until finally you find out that you were in this way unable to control the thoughts generated in your mind. For thousands of years seers have known that thought unaided cannot possibly regulate thought.

It is common knowledge that a person in jumping down from a height or on striking a hammer blow has his mind completely devoid of thought. Intense incidents of this kind produce high tension in the muscles involved, which signals the hypothalamus to curb the thought process. Putting this fact to use, masters of yoga and of the sitting meditation known as *Zazen* train their students to work their respiratory muscles effectively. Learning to initiate and maintain tension in those muscles, the wakefulness center is aroused, and by that means wandering thoughts are inhibited—all while staying fully alert and maximally attentive. Zazen masters developed breathing methods aimed at reaching a steady state of wakefulness with full release of one's potential spiritual energy. Breathing is a singularly uncommon process; it combines the involuntary with the voluntary and is therefore exceptionally well suited for meditation.

With regard to concentration and controlling one's own thought, the lower abdominal muscles, known in Japanese as the *tanden*, play a dominant role. Japanese sumo wrestlers, American football players, circus performers, and racetrack runners must learn how to coordinate their *tanden* and put it in maximal tension and relaxation at will. Then, and only then, can each master the full concentration required for instant release of the tremendous energy levels needed to dart at the goal.

Whatever field of endeavor we choose to engage in, in order to do our best, we must concentrate. The ability to concentrate is a dictate of the will—not a matter of the intellect. Will is the expression of man's spiritual essence, spiritual power if you will. Our energy reserves, awesome as they are, are under direct spiritual control. Intellect doesn't penetrate that vast esoteric domain. Through integrating our physical and spiritual activity, we can harness the major portion of our total capacity—our latent potential. the dormant component. Metaphorically, the eye of my mind sees it like this: an invisible slumbering giant locked underground by an unseeing dwarf. Long since, the dwarf has forgotten what has happened, denies the story, and has lost the key to the cellar, the home of the sleeping giant. We dwarfs of the world must *realize*; to realize is to grow up to full human stature. By and large, we go about utilizing only 10 to 20 percent of our total ability. What a waste!

Where, then, to find the key? Concentration shows the way. Wandering thoughts disrupt concentration and divert attention, delivering us to dead ends. Concentration ploughs through time while harvesting the present, embracing every moment and extracting its juices, its essence—the fragrance of life. Breathe in the *now*; inhale the freshness of time. With concentration, time moves from the abstract to the real, becomes perceptible to our alerted senses. We get to know it, so to speak.

> Say hello to Summer . . .
> Oh, is it Autumn already?
> Does it matter?[1]

The fact that thought unaided cannot control thought is already established. It is here that our physical component ought to be brought into the picture, voluntarily recruited to unite its unique resources with those of the wandering mind.

Physical activity plays an important role in monastic life and is highly valued in many religious sects. It imports an air of harmony and a sense of equanimity. A good many religious communities assign different manual tasks to their members: farming, gardening, pounding grain, digging ditches, preparing meals, etc. None of these duties is frowned upon or considered menial and degrading. Masters, disciples, and would-be disciples chip in. No one is exempt.

In his monastery, Nansen, the great Zen master, carried on his daily chores with liveliness and orderly enthusiasm. Growing old, the master remained dependable, thoroughgoing and

1. From the author's poem "Does it matter?"

amiable. When he showed signs of frailty, his faithful disciples voiced concern, but good old Nansen wouldn't budge; he joyfully continued his daily routine. Worried for his safety, the pupils hid his gardening tools. In response, the master refrained from eating: No working, no eating, he declared. Beset with the risk of starvation, his loving disciples gave in. Happily the master returned to work.

A Zen master once exclaimed, "What is more wonderful than this: I carry water and fetch fuel." "When hungry I eat, when tired I sleep," uttered another master; and "Every day is a good day," declared another. While tending the monastary's backyard, Nansen pointed to a flower and protested, "People of these days see this flower as though they were in a dream."[2] Sounds familiar! "As though they were in a dream"! "We're here now, and this is it," said the bus conductor to Wonderland's dreaming Alice.

> At Nantai I sit quietly with an incense burning,
> One day of rapture, all things are forgotten,
> Not that mind is stopped and thoughts are put away,
> But that there is really nothing to disturb my serenity.[3]
> —Shou-an

2. Katsuki Sekida, *Zen Training* (New York: Weatherhill, 1975), p. 173 et seq.

3. D. T. Suzuki, *Essays in Zen Buddhism, First Series* (New York: Grove Press, 1978), p. 349.

The Interdependence of Body and Mind: Bioenergy

CERTAINLY THE IDEA IS NEITHER NEW NOR UNIQUE, and no single authority can claim credit for discovering that, normally, body and mind interact, influencing one another. In the field of psychotherapy though, Wilhelm Reich, initially a disciple of Freud, fully realized the great significance of such an interdependence. Like some other remarkable disciples of Freud, Reich dared to differ with his mentor. He espoused the Eastern philosophical concept of bioenergy as a pulsatile, harmonious wave diffusing throughout the entire body. He keenly observed the physical manifestations of emotional disorders and carefully monitored their subtle progression into specific bodily attitudes. According to him, those peculiar postures act as barriers, blocking the free flow of bioenergy. He duly labeled them ''character armor.'' Consequently, therapy should be aimed at breaking the individual's armoring to restore the free flow of bioenergy. ''Body work'' became the basis for a number of approaches designed to cure emotional disturbances.

Taking a good look at ourselves, it won't be long before we realize that our postures (muscular patterns), the ways we move about, and many of our muscle aches and tensions correlate with our innermost thoughts and feelings to a considerable degree. Body language expresses the unspoken mysteries of the psyche—distinctive clues that a perceptive eye doesn't overlook.

In targeting the body or the psyche with the appropriate modes of therapy, the desired changes in one or the other will eventually come about. Yoga is an outstanding example of the application of body disciplines to compose and pacify the psyche. Unity of mind and body is a basic tenet of a great many schools of philosophy in the Near, Middle, and Far East.

Nowadays in the West, the notion of "movement therapy" is steadily gaining acceptance. Rudolph Laban and Irmgard Bartenieff[1] believe that body movement in general serves the dual purpose of function and expression. For this reason, a therapist's reach to a patient is a dynamic one—that of body movement. The goal is to establish unity between the physical being, his or her emotional state, and the outside environment—all becoming one. The patient is thereby promoted from a pitiful couch-bound apathetic entity to a lively creature, an active partner sharing with the therapist in finding out the solutions to his or her predicament.

Unfortunately, Freudian casualties still continue to surface, their utter helplessness testifying to the shortcomings of many of Sigmund Freud's theories and assertions. With this in mind, the stressed and depressed ought to say Yes to hope and then arise. "Every moment you are creating yourself. . . . Every moment we are changing the aspect of our existence. . . . This moment is like a switch point on a railway track, of which you have free use. You can switch from an evil course to a good one, and vice versa. Everything depends on your behavior now."[2] Thus there is no good excuse to be negative or cynical, no good reason to gravitate into the bottomless pit. And if you have already sunk in, climb out: there is always a ladder waiting for those who muster the will to ascend in order to reclaim the real self.

1. Irmgard Bartenieff and D. Lewis, *Body Movement: Coping with the Environment* (New York: Gordon & Breach, 1980).
2. Katsuki Sekida, *Zen Training* (New York: Weatherhill, 1981), p. 123.

The Mood of the Meadows:
"Everything Depends on Your Behavior Now"

—Katsuki Sekida, *Zen Training*

THE TIME IS RIPE FOR A JOYFUL WALK. LET US JOIN
Onisura, the poet of Japan. Lovely echoes of his *haiku* happily
sweeten the air; let us tune in:

> How cool the breeze!
> The sky is filled with voices—
> Pine and cedar trees.

If dancing turns you on, go: dance . . . dance! Every time we
dance, it is our first dance. In this spirited moment, I feel rejuvenated by the refreshing embrace of a gentle ocean breeze,
and I hear the sensational sound of the big band proclaiming
the feast of the present. Brave cosmic drums are heartbeating.
Magic flutes inhaling the wind, breathing out songs of continuity. Six lonely guitar strings touched by anonymous feeling hands divulging secret verses long engraved on a human
heart. The trumpet is calling: Come along, all and everyone;
behold the now, the only fragment of life you and I surely have.
Let us dance, each making his or her own dance, capturing the
subtle rhythm of life, smiling, rejoicing, and praising the goodness of the day.

Our individual "character armor" that has shackled us for
so long—shake it loose, let it break, let it shatter. Heavenly
tunes dancing all around—permit them to come through. Let
them revive parts of the body and soul gone numb and dry.
Music's magic power will soon take command, and effortlessly
we will be dancing gaily, softly gliding round and around, merrily hopping up and down like the sprightly, happy child *that
once was you*, or like that certain transient butterfly that one

71

beautiful day got hold of your attention and earned your lavish praise. To self-apprehension, to egocentricity, wave goodbye—not au revoir, nor auf wiedersehen. Instead: *Don't come back!*

Now you are not dancing alone; you *are* the dancing circle, the music, and the dance. In a memorable rhapsody of that kind, a dervish once exclaimed, "This is not my body, this is the Temple of God." Pity, pity, we don't dance as often as we could and should. Our body is bound, our soul is restrained, our will is fettered.

Children dance well before they talk well. *Los Niños*, a De Grazia painting of a children's dance, radiates spontaneity, cheer, motion, and life. *The Rose Dance*, another work of De Grazia, enforces the uplifting message. You see, even for the mortal human body it is most *im*mortal to dance. If we do, it will do us good and import to our world an air of elegant joy.

More to Bees than
Wax and Honey

BEES DANCE, SPIDERS DANCE, BIRDS, FISH, AND MAM-
mals all dance. To charm or entice a would-be mate they dance,
to transmit information or relay a message they dance. Bees
are great dancers; fascinatingly professional, if you will. Circling and wagging are but two of their well-known classics. Circling, they tell other bees: food is near the hive. Wagging says:
it is further away—at a distance of more than 250 feet. Karl
von Frisch took bees seriously; they preoccupied him for several
years. Other intriguing aspects of animal behavior interested
him and became subjects of his research. Into the treasury of
our knowledge Karl von Frisch deposited pearls of information
on bees, fish, and some other wonderful creatures as well. In
appreciation, he was awarded the Nobel Prize for physiology
in 1973.

Several noted anthropologists find ample reason to believe
that dance may have been humankind's first method of com-
munication, predating even the spoken word. To many tribes
of ancient times, dancing was an indispensable ritual function
of their social, religious, and political structure. In spellbinding scenes they danced when capturing a prey; on defeating an
enemy, they danced out their euphoria and gratitude to gods
that loved them and cared. When cruel droughts struck, rain-
dancers pleaded with gods of mercy to soften and bless the earth.
To this day in Africa, the United States of America, and several
other parts of the world, certain communities live by the old
ritual and continue to practice their tribal traditions. They still
dance, praying for rain.

Pharaohs, Pygmies, and
Asian Delicacies

WHILE BUSY CREATING AN IMMORTAL CIVILIZATION, the ancient Egyptians did not neglect the dance. As a matter of fact, we owe them our earliest written records on dancing. The death and rebirth of the god Osiris inspired some of their most elaborate choreography. A religious ceremony in ancient Egypt couldn't possibly be complete without the spiritual disciplines and the touching graces of dance. For their dancing delight the Pharaohs spared no effort. They brought pygmies from Africa and dainty dancing girls from places as remote as India and some other parts of Asia.

From ancient Egypt, the eternal light of art and science traveled to Greece by way of a rugged, significant island: Crete. Believing in the principle of a sound mind in a sound body, the ancient Greeks also took dancing to heart. They danced and danced with enviable enthusiasm. Plato's ideal republic saves a respectable place for the dance in pursuit of "noble, harmonious, and graceful attitudes."

The Show Goes On

IN BOTH EAST AND WEST PEOPLE DANCE, WHILE TUNES vary and movements and methods differ. Western dancers accent footwork. Easterners invite the entire body to the dance, with footwork maintaining rhythm, their whole body emitting poise and mystical beauty. The head, neck, and hand in delicate sequential motion spin an enchanting world of subtleties. Hindu and Bali dancers reached the acme, creating an intriguing spectrum of captivating dancework. Evermore, up to this day, their inspired work delights, fascinates, and baffles even the experienced professional observer.

The *Bharata Natya-Shastra*, a 2000-year-old manuscript of Hindu dance, details numerous movements of different parts of the body. Incredibly, more than 4000 patterns of hand movement, known as *mudras*, have been described. Mudras tell stories, unveil myth, interpret fairy tales, sketch puzzles, and talk prayers. Knowing fingers portray lotus flowers, fishes, fire, desire, gratification, supplication, aggression, conception, remorse for having done wrong, hope, defeat, transport, and overjoy.

Dancers of the Japanese *Kabuki* theater and Western ballet in well-rehearsed movements and gestures magnificently display to their audience the regal elegance of the swan, the astounding beauty of the human body surrendered to art, the undying passions of love, fear, jealousy, sacrifice, anticipation, dream, and desire. Creative dance is gaining popularity and becoming part of the curriculum in a steadily growing number of schools. Children are taught that body language is a form of expression; when appropriate, conversing in movement, with no restraint by preset rules, can be healthy and eloquent.

There isn't a more exhilarating scene than that of dervishes dancing. It's a heavenly delight. Sufist Murshid Samuel L.

Lewis, in his *Spiritual Dance and Walk*, condensed the dervishes' dance scene thus: "The watcher is the prayerful devotee, but the dancer becomes divine." Still, a writer's prose or a poet's verse can only allude to—but never truly interpret or by a long shot reproduce—the magic dimensions of the immortal dervishes' dance.

Out of Its Cocoon:
The Butterfly Rides the Wind

THE DANCE OF THE ANGELS YOU AND I MAY DANCE.
Of angels, how very little we know; so of butterflies let us chat
and gossip.

Once its cocoon breaks open, the butterfly takes off, flying
away—no ifs, no buts, no self-doubt. All preparation for the
flight has been completed in its chrysalis stage. Released, the
butterfly rides the wind. It is in its deepest nature to fly; so
being true, being faithful, it goes for the sky.

Once upon a time in our life a cocoon snapped open, launch-
ing our giant leap, landing us right in the effervescent sea of
existence. Some of us kept on moving, living life, experiencing the ebb and flow; while the rest spent their energies and
limited time-span vacillating, running back and forth to their
cocoon, hiding, doubting, regretting, or merely wishing. While
running away or taking two steps, one forward and one backward, their forefinger is habitually pointing at fate and circumstance; accusing unpredictable events, others; tricky and unkind, chiding an almighty God who refuses to listen, doesn't
appreciate their big hard-earned church donations, and who
doesn't acknowledge their passionate recitations of His Holy
Book.

For these people in their dilemma, the lure of alcohol, tranquilizers, and hypnotic drugs grows irresistible. Many sadly
drift, eventually overpowered by the double tides of delusion
and error. Naive and helpless, others seek the counsel of advi-
sors, gurus, priests, psychiatrists and ministers, believing that
these "masters" are equipped with rafts that will automatically carry them on a promised dream ride to a wonderland of
renewed longevity, power, bounty, and splendor. There, under a magic spell, the Midas touch will be bestowed upon them,

and lo! whatever they will touch will turn to gold. Pitiful dupes, trading in the great human potential for artificial rainbows.

The highest priest, the most revered minister, the purest sheikh or mullah, the greatest rabbi, the enlightened guru, the celebrated psychiatrist—and for that matter the witchiest witch—cannot confer on us what we lack. Among them, a select few point to the path, the Way, and no more. The path is made by walking. Achieving goals is purely a personal endeavor. Unfortunately, many a trusted counselor mischievously or ignorantly claims a power he or she doesn't have, never did, never will—the awesome power to supply and provide. Matter of fact, their insubstantial shoulders cannot carry us around.

Alas! Truth is too near to be visible—a paradox, generally unrecognized, and a costly one. Out of all we know, the surest way to go is to abandon our cocoon once and for all and let come what may. This requires a *second* giant leap. Unlike the very first, this one is chosen, premeditated. Logic and sound intellect reach such a decision; but the final go-ahead is solely a function of the will. Will alone can muster the fortitude needed to pull oneself together for the sorely needed Second Leap.

Even though You Tie a Hundred Knots—
The String Remains One

—Sufi Poet Jalal al-Din Rumi[1]

A MONK ONCE ASKED ZEN MASTER SHIH-T'OU, A successor to one of Hui-neng's disciples, "What is emancipation?" The master asked him in return, "Who puts you under restraint?" At times, the best answer to a formidable question is an equally formidable question. This one is. Zen masters frequently use this seemingly paradoxical method to open disciples' minds. Master Shih-t'ou diagnosed the predicament as self-inflicted and identified the victim as the culprit.

Whenever we fail or suffer, we dash to figure out what has happened. Cause after cause comes to the inquiring mind; yet in reality, the reason is one, only one. With admirable incisiveness, Rumi put it this way: "Even though you tie a hundred knots—the string remains one." Given yarn, every one of us keeps on tying knots; and while this goes on, the mind's eye sees a web of many strings. This criss-cross mental scene, taken for real, generates confusion and panic. And the prey is caught in the web. Who is the prey? Us. Who spun the ensnaring web? Us.

The process is familiar—ancient as humanity itself—and like an amoeba, it perpetually reproduces itself. Here is what happens: As we go about our daily chores, we encounter the expected and unexpected. Generally, we hail or tolerate the first, cheer, loathe, or dread the second. That is precisely where the problem begins and naturally the logical place to dispose of it:

1. Jal al-Din al Rumi, born in Balkh in present-day Afghanistan, died in 1273. A great—possibly the greatest—Sufi poet, his "Spiritual Couplets" influenced Islamic mystical thought and literature. Shortly after his death, his disciples formed the Mawlawiyah Sufi order, known in the West as the Whirling Dervishes.

by *acceptance*—acceptance of outcomes, all outcomes, whatever they are. Acceptance is not surrender, is not defeat. Recognizing and accepting facts and indicators is victory, an honest, unbiased compass always pointing the right direction.

Planning and effort we can control; results, we cannot. Many elements, myriad events seen and unseen, shape results. In large measure these forces cannot be influenced by us. Given this fact, the cry-babies of the universe must stop their crying and save their passionate tears for their unfulfilled, glorious communion with life, its music, its poetry, and the unforgotten great works of art.

This is easier said than done. There is a habitual reluctance to accept; and from all indications, problems generally do not expire at this early stage, as they should. In both cheer and grief we do not see things as they are. Form catches our attention and occupies our thinking, driving away content and meaning. In the daily matters of living we get drawn to one side or the other. In missing one-half, we end up dealing with half-facts, half-truths, half-lies, half-fantasies, half-loves. Totality is slain, wholeness is amputated. Continual change and transformation, a constant feature of our world, are viewed as inconsistencies. Inconsistencies evoke confusion, apprehension, and become threatening. Driven by the unfavorable winds of internal turmoil, the mind's spinning-wheel keeps on turning, spinning yarn after yarn of misconception and make-believe. The handmade, self-tailored cocoon grows around its maker, thickens, hardens, and with time becomes more difficult to crack. The homespun cocoon is but a metaphor for a tall order of human maladies: sorrow, boredom, jealousy, bias, anger, hate, doubt, aggression, deception, and many more wasting ailments that infect the mind and incarcerate the spirit, derailing and crippling the human potential.

To live life to the brim: a proposition splendid and attractive, yet unrealizable within the confinement of a straight-jacket, even though it is woven by our own uncertain hands. For that matter, it isn't physical space that counts, be it an airy citadel or a cloistered conclave; it is the state of mind that draws the limits of our living quarters. Mountains of concrete, tons of cement, steel beams, high walls may protect the physical being of our loved ones and conceal our material possessions, yet they cannot furnish ease of mind or freedom from worry. Many a king and a queen have told us this, at least in their moments of truthful reflection.

The world's inhabitants are for the most part disguised prisoners, labeled "free," physically wandering about, roaming the earth, riding the oceans and the skies—still, captives, real captives to their fears and disenchantment, dwelling in a state of self-perpetuated unhappiness. Doesn't make a bit of good sense, but true. And why? Anywhere we look, including an unhurried look into our own mirror, we encounter the witless and anxious, the disinclined and distracted. Strained, their restless brains cry for help, their minds ready to explode at the seams. Their looks and doings are deceptive. Noisy but not lively; rushing but not progressing; consuming but not assimilating; looking but not seeing; knowing but not understanding; understanding but not realizing; taking but not giving; full but not content; religious but not spiritual; worshiping but not believing; laughing but not joyful; powerful but insecure; well-built but not well; affluent but deficient; courteous but not polite; polite but not gentle; gentle but not genuine; genuine but not warm; tolerant but unforgiving; forgiving but not forgetting; forgetting but not loving; feeling—but only for themselves.

My friend, this beautiful place is packed with wrecks of good men and women pitifully gone to the bad. "Who put them under restraint?" "Who tied the knots?" The dungeon in which we languish is erected by our own foolish hands. Brick by brick, with every trial or unexpected event, the sinister walls rise, open windows grow fewer, gates get heavier and move slower and slower. What, eventually, is left of the Universe? A cocoon with a peephole through which the view is narrow, bleak, dim. And back to the cocoon, there goes Homo sapiens! Alas!

Instead, we should be moving toward uncontaminated childhood, where it all began—to our original, pure Self before we got twisted into our present complaining forms, before the arrival of heavy clouds of misconception, hangups, and petty rationalizations. Lest this sound cynical or despairing, it is not to give up hope. Our present dark shadow still bears a light spot. We mustn't lose sight of it, must never let it flicker out. Darkness swallows light, light shatters darkness. It isn't the tail-end of the rainbow; it is only the beginning.

Forever—for every moment of time—there is a new rainbow, a second chance, another option, a fresh opportunity. The shock of recognition may come as a tidal wave, may knock us flat down, but among us some will always rise, stand their ground, say Yes and make it happen. On the pathways of recovery, we will reclaim our former innocence, courage, innate freedom, spontaneity, and creativity. Freed, we will wave goodbye to stress and sorrow. A new stature will have arisen.

I Took Her for a Swan

TO REGAIN OUR NATURAL FREEDOM, TO RECAPTURE the rhythm of time and the tempo of life, many of us must endure a training period and accept certain basic disciplines. Training period! Certain disciplines! Ugh! *Whyyy?* Aren't we adults? This may have the ring of the unreasonable and the condescending; it may even seem some sort of undeserved penalty. Not at all. Far from it. It is merely a reorganization of one's inner workings, a resetting, necessary and overdue. If you wish, you may refer to it as a therapeutic measure, tried and known to work. And in all fairness, the pill isn't all that bitter and hard to swallow. Its aftertaste is actually quite sweet and mellow.

The human mind being impressionable and conditioned, therefore to relearn the right way, we must unlearn the acquired straying, wasteful ways. And, we cannot have it both ways and expect to make it and be happy and secure. "The great way is easy, yet people prefer by-paths" says the *Tao Te Ching*. Arts and sports confirm the wonders that regular training and good discipline can bring about, reactivating the idle body and rekindling the spark of the inert spirit. The high destination of arts and sports is the restoration of freedom to the human mind, breaking loose its artificial restraints, letting its glory and awesome potential unfold.

An open free mind thinks what it feels, feels what it thinks, and brings to unity a physical body loosened and brought back to its former elegance. With mind and body attuned, spontaneity and freshness will lift the state of siege, dispelling unease, boredom, and self-doubt. On this rearranged stage, work and play—the only two things we do—transform into fulfilling experiences, each feeding on the other and propelling it along a continuum of adequacy and harmony. In this firmament, the seeds of stress fail to germinate.

In pursuit of self-liberation and fulfillment, Eugen Herrigel, a German professor of philosophy, took an unusual step: breaking the barrier by means of perfection of the art of archery. The path he walked was six years long in—where else?—the land of Zen, samurai, and the rising sun: Japan. The philosophy master willingly submitted his whole lot to the caring hands of another master, no ifs, no buts, no looking backward. In a skinny manuscript,[1] he portrayed the memorable experience. His narrative flows like a clear mountain spring. The sincere reader is rewarded with much to think about, much to feel, a whole spectrum to quietly contemplate.

" 'The right shot at the right moment does not come because you do not let go of yourself. You do not wait for fulfillment but brace yourself for failure,' the Japanese master roared." On another occasion while observing Herrigel's practice, the master commented:

> Your arrows do not carry because they do not reach far enough spiritually. You must act as if the goal were infinitely far off. For master archers it is a fact of common experience that a good archer can shoot farther with a medium-strong bow than an unspiritual archer can with the strongest. It does not depend on the bow, but on the presence of the mind. In order to unleash the full force of this spiritual awareness, you must perform the ceremony differently, rather as a good dancer dances. . . . dance and dancer are one and the same. By performing the ceremony like a religious dance, your spiritual awareness will develop in full force.

Towards the end, Herrigel mastered the art of self-forgetfulness and could then transcend technique. His art became "an artless art growing out of the unconscious."

1. Eugen Herrigel, *Zen in the Art of Archery* (New York: Vintage Books, 1971), pp. 33, 62.

From the sublime art of archery to the whimsical art of synchronous swimming; from an adroit philosophy professor to a quaint, dainty swimmer—Tracy Ruiz. Her unforgettable performance during the 1984 Los Angeles Summer Olympics aroused a waning interest in a fanciful sport and won her a gold medal. I take delight in recalling her. That warm day in August, with the music softly playing, with the velvet paws of a cat, Tracy danced her steps to the swimming pool . . . paused for a moment or two (my guess: a prelude to the necessary ritual of self-detachment) . . . then lovingly offered herself to the yielding water.

No splashes, no ripples—only the harmonious wave of a great embrace charged the still air. Happy to be together, the water and the muse; a spell interwoven of music, dance, dancing mermaid, and aquatic stage, all imperceptibly transformed into one breathtaking scene. A knowledgeable source said that the champion swimmer had been dancing under water several hours every day for no less than 11 years. Here, then, is yet another fascinating example of "artless art growing out of the unconscious." (Incidentally, Tracy is extraordinarily beautiful. I took her for a swan.)

The subconscious; the mysterious lush caverns of the human mind where the vast portion of our best experience and knowledge is deposited. A treasure-trove in waiting, rarely tapped, ever broadcasting signals, speaking codes and sending clues, trying to link with the world of the conscious mind. Yet one's self-consciousness stands in the way, ignoring the subconscious and slamming the door. In its attempt to bridge the gap between the conscious and subconscious, human experience time and again has confirmed the futility of voluntary recall. It isn't the right key for unlocking the door. Paradoxical as it may seem, self-effacement—in other words, self-detachment—happens to be the key leading to magic regions within which our larger composition is orchestrated. Regrettably, many never hear their own best composition.

Practically speaking, it isn't an easy matter to disengage from one's own self. "Oh dear!" is the usual response whenever such a proposition is raised. Sounds weird, like taking off for an extended leave of absence only to get lost in the stratosphere. Who wants to be part of that? Where is the return ticket? Well, there is nothing for nothing. To grow and become what we dream and cherish, we must expand beyond the insubstantial constraints of one's individual self and experience the roomy ambience of the Higher Self. The Higher Self is not a mysterious ghost or an alien master or a fictitious character. It is us, the real us, the human essence, the vital force perpetually and miraculously flowing from the infinite source, seeding and flourishing in every one of us, re-creating, reproducing, echoing notes to the tunes of which we toil, wonder, rise or fall.

To the blind stare of self-delusion, the "tableau vivant" is infinitely far, a Fata Morgana, unreal, at best unreachable, save perhaps for the prophets and saints. Yet in truth it is a commonwealth, real, attainable, always available and infinitely close. It is but the boundless sphere within; it is our core, the flowering meadows of infinite choices we can choose from, the inexhaustible options we can exercise, the capacity to say Yes or No, to do or to refrain, to feel or to grow numb, to think or to reflex, to view the world through our tears or through joyful anticipation.

At the boundary line, a little bit beyond, the strangling cord of circumstance snaps off, the confining walls of the individual ego tumble down, and the tugs of opposites break loose. The ticket of admission is self-knowledge through self-discipline, regular practice of some sort of meditation, and restoration of one's ability to concentrate deeply.

The reborn human perceives and recognizes the revelations of the subconscious mind, welcomes the nascent images, listens to verses coming into being, harnesses tunes beginning to form, nurtures thoughts gently moving about, follows the twinkling bud of light, and reverberates to palpitations emanating from all other forms of life. The reborn human handles all in deep affection, unruffled, content, cuddles them reverently in the

86

labyrinth of the conscious mind, calmly contemplates the promising broods, tends the newly born sprouts, joyfully flirts with the blooms, dancing, adding, erasing, laughing, clowning, and compassionately performing each task. Such is the methodology of the noble geniuses among us. In them we admire and envy the greatness that crosses our path. But, insecure and lazy, we let it go, slipping away between the numb fingers of our hesitant hands.

Art and Liberation:
A Brave Page

IN GRANDEUR AND SPLENDOR, THE WORLD OF ENTERtainment displays some of our best aspects—elegance, tenderness, cheer, and passion—its presentation real and allegorical, portraying what the human spirit, once liberated, is capable of putting out. On the enchanting stage, the show is nonetheless *for real*. There, when the lights dim and the curtain goes up, the mind's viewing eye recognizes our unfulfilled yearnings, our reasonable and unreasonable dreams, our brief and not-so-brief frustrations, the tormenting sense of guilt, the longing for the promised redemption, uncured hang-ups, memories of our former innocence, hide-and-seek (child and adult versions), undanced steps, unsung songs, heaven as we see it, the hell we know and the hell we dread, passional tears, tears to get by and "don't forget!" as well as those certain tears that never come out and the raw spots that keep aching every so often.

Makeup, colors, costumes, motion, and music regale our eager senses. But great performers do not pretend. In royal armor, under a clown's hat, in a harlot's tunic, among the swans, they willingly surrender their identity; with ease and grace they break away to live and relive their roles, more regal than a king, funnier than a clown, more bedizened than a harlot—and with the poise, elegance, and stateliness of a swan. Heroes and villains, masters and beggars, martyrs and executioners of all times reborn on the stage; revived by the creative touch of the art.

In talking with reporters about the legendary James Brown, renowned as "Soul Brother Number One," a fan of his once said, "James Brown is magic. . . . the man gets out of himself, . . . he's got a kind of freedom. I crave it. Every day." *Gets out of himself*—a brief statement, casual, yet intuitive and profound. Slipping out, so to speak, smoothly detaching from the rigmarole and the tightening grip of oneself. The barrier of habit and convention limiting modern man and woman as never before must be penetrated, and everyone must do it on his or her own. No one can penetrate the barrier on behalf of someone else. No one can deliver or redeem but oneself. Claims to the contrary are false, serving only to perpetuate apathy and foster dependency. Apathy and dependency may readily convert to anxiety and hostility.

With the barrier broken, new, unlimited horizons appear—I should say *recognized*, for the so-called new horizons aren't really new; they have been there all the time. The human microcosm, limited in itself, cannot grow to expectation without embracing the whole Universe—the macrocosm. But where is the meeting point for the great embrace? And when? Everywhere, anywhere, and at any time. Incomplete, shouldn't we try to retrieve what has been missing? Incomplete, how can we safely navigate the ocean of circumstance and reclaim true liberation?

A question that challenges the human intellect and subdues the will to freedom is: Can we "slip out" with our feet still touching the familiar ground? Our jobs and means of making a living—will they remain secure? Our dear relations, our loved ones—will they wait for us? Well, why not? The trail of liberation trod by the artist, the poet, the sage, and many not-so-famous proves that the fear of self-liberation is unfounded. The travelers haven't gotten lost; they kick around longer and glow brighter than most.

Fear is uncalled for. Fear, after all, of what? And wherefore? We are not inanimate feathers drifting in the wind. We are not shipwrecks driven ashore by the forces of some sea. The human organism will always instinctively gravitate to the human colony and will find its way back. Nature, art, intuition, cleared-out intellect, and the indomitable human will—none is alien to us; each *is* us—will secure our points of reference, keep us human, and save us from getting lost in oblivion.

At this point a brave page confirming art's noble role in freeing body and spirit ought to be revealed. Throughout history, the human consciousness has witnessed the dance and heard the song of its oppressed and dispossessed. Trampled down and experiencing the taste and aftertaste of sorrow, they carve with song and dance an outlet, a spiritual refuge, saving them from the dead life of despair and slow decay. Their unrehearsed music, dance, and folklore come out pure and natural. Lacking the gigantic dimension of the classical symphony, devoid of contemporary orchestral complexity, their compositions are lean and haunting.

More like the quickening heartbeat of a racetrack runner, the peristaltic undulations of a dancing goddess, the long-hoped-for rigors of hibernation coming to an end, difficult breathing under imminent threat, the rustle of leaves telling of the wind's path and strength, the nocturnal howl of the wolf, the flapping of eagles' wings, and the memory of rain—stomping, clapping, chanting, or singing in pantomime—their overtures are forceful and tempestuous. They've ''got rhythm''; their tempo is that of the season and the hour; their melody speaks of the beast, the human, the earthly, the divine, and of the unsettled fate of man. No, it isn't tears, it isn't wailing; it isn't laughter; it isn't prayers, either. It is all of that . . . and more.

The masters of the mansion—full, bored, restless, drinking all the wine, shuffling all the cards, crowding all the ballrooms, ever looking for more diversions; taking time, always finding time, killing time, with plenty of time: the masters don't need much ear to hear the primal notes. The tide is forceful. The masters are drawn in, pulled by an unseen, unbreakable current that links human souls, all souls, all sentient souls. They applaud, they cheer, they envy. But it isn't cheer, admiration, or jealousy that brought out the song and dance. The oppressed and the dispossessed can't help it. How long can a volcano contain its wrath and flames? Can an ocean rein in its surf?

When living matter is injured or restrained, it senses and reacts. Its energy wave unties the tongue, fiddles resting vocal

90

cords, launches a whole vocabulary of movements, raw and graceful, meaningful and thunderous, steeped in tenderness and other subtle emotions not to be told. This is black magic, gypsy magic, the wanderer's spell, the haunting tapestry of the underdog. A live brew, ingredients tart to bitter, spicy to caustic; tinder sparks, dynamite; all universal and human. What about the leftovers? What about the aches, the rancor, the ashes? Where are: the tormented flesh, the tired bones, the bare nerve endings, the sweat, the stink, the tears? *Jazz, calypso, flamenco,* and *the blues.* In their diaries, literate aristocrats allude to the tragedy in trivial footnotes: it isn't art, after all; it is merely the habitual weepings of unweaned children, premature ejaculations of restless adolescents, carnival frenzies, spirituals—all unworthy. A postscript will do.

> Hold your tongue, hold your tongue,
> Because I have hidden things about you,
> Little secrets that no one knows.
> All black eyes
> Are to be taken prisoner tomorrow.
> Yours are so black
> You must cover your face with a veil.
>
> —Flamenco song

Flamenco is a moving glory of Andalusian magic. Under the tyranny of the Inquisition, the outcast gypsies, Muslims, and Jews of Spain entrusted their anguish, despair, horror, faith, and love to the tempest-like dance. From dark violet to flaming red, the scene moves from the *soleares* (serious) to the *alegrias* (light), with different shades reduced to mildness or given raging intensity. Rainbow renditions, spellbinding and compelling. Folk songs are flamenco's essence, guitar its music. Hand-clapping, finger-snapping, admiring shouts, castanets, and jingling tambourines add a special touch and zesty spice to the immortal dance.

Men, manly—assertive and notoriously proud—click their toe and heel with primal masculinity, improvising while they dance. The female magnet steps in, casting the bait, affirming the exquisite grace of hand and body motion. At the rending of the veil, their body is returned to them and their soul is revealed. The *fandangos grandes, farruca, malagueñas, cartageñeras, bulerías* continue to tell and charm. (Yet with commercial interests infesting the arts, rehearsed routines are alarmingly jeopardizing and replacing spontaneity.)

Blues, jazz, flamenco, and similar works of art are unsolicited testimonials—unauthorized quivering of the heart chambers, full, aspiring to pump out their secrets before grim rigor mortis stills them. Caught in the magic yarn, masters and conquerors are overcome. Tunes and rhymes they instigated gain momentum and acquire power of their own. Here we are: again and again, the hunters are hunted, the master's iron fist grows numb and loose. An exchange of shackles. With the undaunted power of art, the slaves and outcasts who couldn't read or write letters could dictate and rhapsodize.

Wounded brothers and sisters, wherever you are: take heart. Your brave trumpet will silence the gun, your fearless drum will subdue the whip; your dance, your freedom ballads, your "let-me-out" songs, and why-must-it-be verses will enlist others and will embrace and ensnare your oppressors. Hold on! The lines of life, hope, and love will always endure. History books tell. Readers of history: Beware!

Look what they have done to the story; here are some of their unedited interpretations and conclusions: "Such are the examples of lofty, noble revolutions . . . Detestable savagery perpetrated by a fugitive bunch of barbarians . . . Liberation movements . . . Terrorist acts threatening decent peace-loving industrialized nations . . . Rightful execution of war criminal . . . Justifiable self-defense . . . Serves our own interests, our friends' and allies' . . . Hot pursuit of criminal gangs . . . Preemptive strikes to prevent future strikes . . . War to prevent war." The scene is one; yet one cries foul, the other sings praises.

More and more I distrust historians, I loathe history books. Narrating the same happening, scripts widely diverge and the truth gets slayed in between. The louder voice reaches the press, gets coverage by the news media, and carries the day. The truer account of the story I increasingly search for in novels and veiled lyrics. One needs to reach beneath the mask, though, and unravel the plot.

The Keynote of Nature:
"Everything Depends on Your Behavior Now"

—Katsuki Sekida, *Zen Training*

THE SOUND OF A RIVER, THE ROAR OF THE SEA, THE
rustle of treetops in a large forest, the noise of a large city on
one's threshold—all have a certain tone with a definite pitch.
Professors Rice and Silliman, cited in *The Voice of the Silence*,
define this tone as the middle F of the piano scale. An interesting scientific finding, this which is thrown at us; what shall
we do with it? Knowing isn't enough. What counts is the realization, the personal experience. "Everything depends on your
behavior now."

In tuning in to nature, acknowledging its splendors, listening to its pacifying notes, peace, quiet recollection, and ability to concentrate deeply come our way. Remaining aloof and
withdrawn, a penalty comes instead: boredom, stress, and
depression. Eventually, isolation and a life in exile. Spiritual
exile.

Watching a bird in flight—attentively, not with a casual
glance or a disinterested, cursory look; unhurriedly following
the flight path, carefully noting the movement of the wings,
the overlapping feathers, the graceful turn of the head, neck,
and beak, the high soar and the gentle, soft glide without loss
of altitude: with our pictorial perception of the bird's flight continuing, an inner feeling of lifting-up, unloading, so to speak,
is transmitted to us.

A good bird-watcher senses my meaning here. In such a com-
pliant state, mind yields its rigid framework, contingencies and
circumstance take a back seat, their magnitude scales down,
their sharp cutting edge blunts. The turbulent atmosphere
calms down and all will be viewed in the new serene light. Sur-
prising how a slight alteration of mental mood can induce major
changes in seeing and perceiving! Birds in flight have always

inspired some of our happiest lyrics—many a great musical composition, scientific discoveries, and inventions as well. "Free as a bird" expresses a joyous human/bird interlude, a dialogue meant to endure within a desirable state of mind.

On an early morning as you open your window to dawn, say good morning to the first birds, pay attention as they call, watch them flying out of their nests to travel the high roads of the air. Often the eager wings of an early bird bring to the human eye the twinkling light of the sun's very first rays. Blessed are those who witness the rebirth of the day. It does them good, plenty of good. The very first sun-rays, a bird's eager wings, and the early-morning riser are all in a certain sense one.

Roses and other flowers, pleasant, living quietly in themselves "without a why," good-natured, their fragrance sweetening the air—every season they return. For whom? Recognizing the pleasant, we will become pleasant. Beholding the beautiful, we will be beautiful. Observing serenity, we will realize serenity. Seeking harmony, we will receive harmony. Searching for the peaceful, we will have peace. Helpful transformations! With continued practice they are bound to happen to us. One's mental attitude and commitment determine the "if" and the "when."

We are the five senses: seeing, hearing, touching, smelling, and tasting—with a mind interpreting and sorting out. If input is amiable and worthwhile, so the output will be. Recalling the computer buzzword GI:GO (garbage in: garbage out), it's up to us to straighten the equation and improve the output. *Goodness in, goodness out; truth in, truth out; cheer in, cheer out; compassion in, compassion out;* all of them workable propositions worth considering and implementing. Dwelling in conflict and joining ranks with the crude and vulgar, we become quarrelsome, course, and lacking. Surely we can rise and become the person we long to be. The choice is ours.

Begin now, listen to the raindrops falling on your window sill, the sound of the ocean retold by the seashell you are holding to your ear. Witness a red moon just before dawn; moonlight in September; Venus glittering in the western sky; a tree

95

reflected in a pond; clouds in transit; rainbows making brief appearances; a master weaver, the spider, mending its web; a snail out of its shell on an errand—soft, slow, and clever. An old woman on a cane taking her two dogs for a stroll. A lonesome old man adopting a stray cat. Someone in the park feeding the geese and the pigeons. Two children holding hands. Delightful encounters.

Behold for a while; a little may rub off here and there. Fellowship with nature sharpens our senses, renews our energy, and multiplies our productivity. "Making it" with nature, our mood becomes less moody, our countenance more becoming, our thinking more thoughtful, organized, and inclined to the positive. Our whole being endures better, tolerates more, and willingly adapts to what comes along. On this plane, we become "unassailable"; nothing can disturb our harmony, everything is seen as it really is and placed in proper relationship with other things, all being interdependent and interconnected. Work and play will merge, become one, and whatever we do will come out very well. Time spent with nature is not wasted, and the race is not always to the swift.

Slow me down, Lord!
Ease the pounding of my heart by the
quieting of my mind.
Steady my hurried pace,
With a vision of the eternal reach of time.
Give me, amidst the confusion of my day,
The calmness of the everlasting hills.
Break the tension of my nerves
With the soothing music of the singing streams
That live in my memory.
Teach me the art of taking minutes,
vacations of slowing down,
To look at a flower;
To chat with an old friend or make
a new one;

To pat a stray dog; or to watch a spider
build a web;
To smile at a child; or to read a good book.
Remind me each day
That the race is not always to the swift;
That there is more to life
Than increasing its speed.

—Orin L. Crane

Astronomers and physicists deciphered many a mystery of the Universe while quietly and patiently observing the sky above, the passing of time, night and day, the four seasons, stars glittering, the eclipses, the solar and lunar cycles, the direction of the wind, birds flying against the wind, lightning preceding echoes of thunder, clouds on the run, objects falling down and shadows expanding and contracting. Scientists and philosophers of Ancient India, Egypt, Iran, China, and Mexico precisely defined the cosmos, the galaxies, the solar system, the shape of the earth, and the duration of the years. Equipped with powerful telescopes and highly sophisticated tools, modern scientists came later on, adding some and confirming most. "We are like dwarfs seated on the shoulders of giants; we see more things than the ancients and things more distant, but this is due neither to the sharpness of our own sight nor to the greatness of our stature, but because we are raised and borne aloft on that giant mass."[1]

Respect for all cultures, past and present, will keep us humble, decent, and fair. We owe chemistry, physics, mathematics, algebra, biology, and many other subjects to a few men and women who dared to raise questions, wonder, and wander. Their minds open, their spirits free, they explored the earth, the sea, the nature of objects, motion, the hot, the still, the

1. Bernard of Chartres, the twelfth-century French humanist and philosopher. Quoted in J. B. Ross and M. M. McLaughlin, *The Indispensable Medieval Reader* (New York: The Book Society, 1950), p. 1.

icy, the inner workings of the human mind, and the miracle of creation. And the crowd? Always busy, very busy, always short of time, always losing time, staying on the receiving end, breathlessly catching the world by its tail.

Have you ever stopped to ask yourself why the fuchsias look down, while tulips look up—? In a vast orchard, a single white flower displaying a thin red streak not observed on the other flowers—how come? Could this be a blemish—or a mark of distinction? Will it hinder or advance its species? Why do wolves and ravens have affinity for each other?[2] We have only two eyes; why not four? Why do the Great Pyrenes and St. Bernards tend to develop a sixth toe on their hind limbs? Among fish, why are only tuna warm-blooded? Why does the bat, a mammal, fly while the ostrich, a bird, doesn't? When certain sponges are pulled apart, their pieces come together again, recovering unity of the whole. Why? These matters invite speculation and inquiry. Exploring them, the mind remains operative and agile.

In attending to nature's animate and inanimate components, we realize their mutual interdependence and appreciate the unique function of each. Getting to know them the way they are, we learn how to coexist with them and even to love them for themselves. At this point, harming or wasting them becomes reprehensible to us. Members of the animal kingdom, forests and what they host, plants, rivers, oceans, natural resources and environment—all will be guarded by the human shepherd and loving guardian rather than plundered by the heartless human brute. Injury, whenever inflicted, harms the victim and debases the perpetrator. In the process, the assailant is always disfigured.

In its myth and grandeur, nature moves the artist, ultimately claiming his whole being. The artist wanders and reflects. Fascinated by the scenes he encounters, he looks them over and over, closer and closer, deeper and deeper. In his heart he experiences their transiency—or he may have to move on, walk

2. The Indians and Eskimos of North America have noted this extraordinary affinity. In their legends the bird and the mammal are frequently coupled.

away. To hold on to the transient, he recreates it on canvas or sketches it on paper, in effect locking or fixing it. Carving a wood block, moulding a shapeless mass of clay, chiseling unshapely stone, dignifying words by making them poems, giving music to the world, it is his way—the artist's way—of holding on to the beautiful and interpreting the compelling. In the process, his work passes on to others; in other words, he propagates the exquisite and gives a touch of permanency to the transient and the temporal.

All this is but one way. It doesn't explain all works of art, but it does answer to some. The artist may not be conscious of all this or of his own reason. At any rate, he can't help it; he does it anyway. What you see is the artist's inside, his soul. But what about the necessary conception, gestation, labor pains, confinement, bewilderment, merriment and humorous interludes? That is for us to figure or dig out. The artist merely hands us what he considers a finished product; yet, all great works of art are in a certain sense *unfinished*.

Fear of Death:
How to Cope with It

Said the serpent to Eve: Death is not an unhappy thing
when you have learned how to conquer it.

—George Bernard Shaw, *Back to Methuselah*

ONE MAN DIES, ANOTHER MAN DIES, BUT MEN DO
not die. A bird succumbs, a second bird succumbs, but birds
will live. A flower withers, another flower withers, but flowers
will always bloom. Haunted by the memory of the man he
killed during the Colombian civil war, Nobel laureate Gabriel
García Marquez's grandfather told him, "You can't imagine
how much a dead man weighs."

I hated death. I feared death. From childhood on, I carried
my hate and fear with me. There, in between my ribs, the two
remained ominously glued to my breast. Mere mention of the
five-letter word automatically triggered discomfort and heartache. The gloomy prospect of ultimate decay added to my trou-
bles. Loved ones kept on leaving, never to return in their lively
human form. Painful experiences all but enforced and legitimized my unhappy state of mind. Tales of ghosts and eyewit-
ness accounts of awesome deeds by wicked spirits poured into
my head.

I was a child then, and the storytellers were respected elders
besides those others one came to like and trust. Growing up,
I took my ghosts with me; as a matter of fact, they refused to
leave me alone and I had to move on, so we kept uneasy company with each other. Along the roads of life they multiplied,
and their shadow seemed to grow bigger.

Of all things, loneliness invited them the most. Darkness,
the sound of thunder, hooting of owls, cheerless dialogues of
somber crows, heartrending yowls of coyotes, mournful howls
of persecuted wolves—all readily raised the curtain on a most

unwelcome cast. In full gear, the unfriendly gang paraded the daunted stage of my mind; quarrelsome, cynical, mean.

Time passed. Childhood ended. Adolescence followed—quick, vigorous, restless. There and then something happened, big and unexpected. Of their own accord, with nothing conscious on my part, these vicious ghosts began to transform—and what a dramatic transformation that was! They seemed to have aged some; their bold, rich colors started fading into austere shades of gray; their enthusiasm and morbid interest in my personal affairs turned into cold indifference. Finally, they ran out of steam and quietly expired.

This, I must admit, surprised me, for I thought ghosts never died. Mine did. The dramatic demise of my childhood ghosts brought a measure of comfort and the prospect of peace to my mind; but somewhere on the horizon, that old unsettling fear of extinction still knocked about.

Of all my experiences with death and dying, one happens to be "decisive" and worth telling. On a pleasant September day, summer was leaving for some other regions of the planet and autumn was on the threshold. The warm spell of dry weather was tempered by a refreshing, balmy breeze that imported distant aromas of roses and jasmines. An early-morning high wind swept the predawn clouds eastward, and the sun presided over a clear blue sky. Birds were everywhere celebrating, and things were falling in their right places, or so it seemed.

My car had driven that stretch of the broad boulevard innumerable times before. Tall trees and shady sidewalks skirted the paved motorway. Blemishing the pretty scene, though, was a vast graveyard that grimly outlined the south side of the boulevard. It seemed out of place. Gravesites ought to stay far away, very far away. They belong to the other world—one that is off limits, at least for me. I kept tombs and corpses out of sight always, or almost always. They spelled grief and sorrow, downers for which I had no use; so I faithfully adhered to my discipline of avoidance.

Eventually, though, time and circumstance break just about

every discipline. On this particular day, mine broke. Here is what happened, all of it still clear in my mind despite the lapse of several years:

Unconsciously my restrained eyes turned left, stealing a timorous glance at the somber landscape. There, under the tall assertive trees, my hesitant eye met a boy and a girl leisurely strolling along the shady sidewalk. They were holding hands, amiably flirting with one another, whispering and giggling, wrapped in the sweet search for love and the promise of happiness that comes with it. They seemed oblivious of the world around. Their affectionate, slow steps claimed the better part of my attention.

Soon I sensed a gentle, happy feeling overcoming me. A new, positively charged wave physically intruded into my negatively charged inner field. Two random forces, mutually opposite, mutually attractive, had come together. Then, within the secret realm of a trespassing, onlooking soul, their embrace instantly sowed the seed of enlightenment that conquers fear and opens the eye of the mind to see things as they are. I reveled in it. My weary senses happily quit their nervous reserve, relishing the dawning of a new light. A spell of ease came along, a pure ease that I had only heard of, read about, and longed for.

My eyes, now unrestrained, freely wandered beyond the sidewalk, crossing over the old boundary line of the cemetery, the forbidden territory of the past. I must have kept gazing at the tombs, all the while driving in the newly found atmosphere—an atmosphere not induced by the calculating and discriminating intellect. This was instead the fruit of a special state, a state where one's whole being transforms into a single receptive unit, pliant, harmonious, open—wide open—permitting this and that to enter freely to find its mate, its so-called opposite. There are no preconditions; everything seeks its natural place, rests contentedly with others without antagonizing or kicking out something else, all in harmonic coexistence with time. In this freedom zone, now my whole being, the traditional mournful interment scene gave birth to another spectacle—one of creation and joy. The two seemed to dance together to a mysterious, eternal tune.

Amazing how so much depends on so little! Strange how we go about afraid and confined; yet an accidental, seemingly trivial event, an unscheduled rendezvous, a passing comment not even meant for us may help trigger a radical change in our temperament and mental attitude. That day, the opened eye of my mind while scanning the land of the dead discovered no fangs, no claws, no daggers, no arrows, no guns, no bombs—bloody tools of destruction, all belonging to the inhabitants of the world out there, the one *outside* the cemetery line. Among the dead, I felt safe. Content? Maybe! In the cemetery, all is calm, profoundly peaceful and still.

In reaching my destination that day—the emergency room of a community hospital serving a densely populated quarter of a big metropolis—I was responding to an emergency call. The despatch was terse and grave. "Doctor, we have an eighteen-year-old male with multiple gunshot wounds of the chest and abdomen. His condition is very critical." I dashed in, galloping right through the hospital's main corridor to the emergency unit where everyone's attention was focused on the mortally wounded youth.

Here was a well-built young man who by all standard medical indicators was much closer to death than to life, yet who by virtue of his youth and apparent past state of health was more fit to live than to die. Pints of blood and other fluids were being pumped into his collapsed veins by diligent nurses while the physician on duty was busy slipping a tube down his throat through which he received artificial respiration by a mechanical ventilator. Too weak, too much in shock even to perform the vital, seemingly effortless, seemingly involuntary task of breathing.

With so much taken for granted, we do not realize how much we have going for us, how much is given us, until loss occurs or seems imminent. How wonderful to be able to inhale and exhale without burden or pain! Take a few moments to contemplate and acknowledge. All the necessities for life's eventful journey are graciously granted from the beginning, the very beginning. Remember.

To come back: with the mechanical respirator breathing for him, the patient stopped thrashing and calmed down some, the premortal blue color of his skin and lips vanishing to reveal an ominous pale complexion of massive blood loss. My examining hands touching his forehead encountered a cold, damp surface, chilling, more like that of a marble tombstone at dawn. His moribund figure resembled a statue of wax; yet three obscene bullet holes located in the front and left side of his trunk—with warm red blood incessantly welling out of them, dreadfully mixed with copious froth—were grim reminders that the figure in question was not of wax. Still alert, his anxious eyes clung to me for life, as if ardently begging for my troops to move in, to do something, real quick, *right now*, to restore his youthful being before it was too late.

In a matter of minutes, the poor soul was lying still, anesthetized, stretched on an operating room table. His heart, lungs, and liver—all indispensable—suffered serious life-threatening injuries. We all fought hard—doctors, nurses, and medical technicians. We were racing against the clock. Through deliberate speed we slowed down the passage of time, thus limiting permanent damage of the mutilated vital organs to a minimum. It took us three hours to do this and to control the devastating hemorrhage. At last our efforts bore fruit, and not long after surgery our young man gained consciousness in the recovery room. We were all elated, looked to one another, and shared a heartfelt sigh of relief. A few hectic days followed, but this patient's strong will to live made a difference, in my opinion. The agony of excruciating pain, nausea, chills, lack of appetite, and extreme frailty did not subdue his spirit. He cooperated with us and did his share. We did ours as well. It was a good partnership. Finally, he walked out the hospital gate, head up, without a crutch, a cane, or any other form of assistance.

As I waved him good-bye, a voice inside me whispered: The

dead, the ghosts, the spirits cannot do us harm. It is the living we have to watch for, it is the living who can do us in, make war or peace, wound or mend, wave an olive branch or point a gun at our head. The city of the dead is calm and quiet, its citizens have long laid down their arms.

The events of this day, though paradoxical and intense, were all pressed within a short period of time—a mere three hours and a few minutes—and yet their impact, meaningful details, tragedy and sobering essence never left my memory. In their aftermath, my own mother's final days came back to mind as an elegy or a substantial footnote with undisguised, perhaps understandably personal, overtones. Years had gone by, and passionate lament had matured into the enduring warmth of remembrance. She and I were very close. In the "twilight zone" before her passing, we both realized and accepted the inevitable. She would not feel lonesome having me by her side, I knew that. I also knew that this indomitable woman had no particular need of my support: her immense personal courage and unshaken faith always took care of her.

She was, then, an undaunted soul whose kidneys had given up on her, with no cure in sight. Love, sympathy, empathy, and family tradition dictated our course of action; so we kept my mother at home with us, in her own bedroom with all her familiar surroundings, everything left undisturbed. Soon thereafter she lapsed into a deep coma; yet moments before death finally struck—as if intent on not disappointing us—she slowly opened her beautiful sleepy eyes, her placid face showing a faint glow reminiscent of the setting sun. A few gasps—irregular, fitful, and shallow—and it was all over. My mother was gone. She had left us. A serene good-bye smile anointed her beautiful face, now stilled, dead silent; but her smile miraculously survived.

Let the world—myself included—sing the praises of Mona Lisa and her smile; but within me, alone, deep—within a special place in my heart—my mother's smile will live. Looking back on my mother's final days, I do not think the angel of death was particularly unkind or harsh on her. On the contrary, I thought that it was thoughtful and gentle. Upon departure she seemed well at ease; content! Like a bird flying south at day's end.

Lewis Thomas wrote in *The Lives of a Cell*: "If you stand in a meadow, at the edge of a hillside, and look around carefully, almost everything you can catch sight of is in the process of dying, and most things will be dead long before you are."[1] On beholding the meadows, Walt Whitman exclaimed: "The smallest sprout tells me there is no death." Overjoyed, the poet added: "I swear I think there is nothing but immortality." The biologist August Weismann pointed out that certain living organisms multiply by splitting into living halves. They never die. Death therefore is neither natural nor inevitable.

It is estimated that planet earth is four and a half billion years old, and it is generally accepted that it took no less than a half billion years for mother earth to deliver its very first offspring, simple living entities: the prokaryotes. Their name is aptly descriptive, *pro* meaning "before" and *karyote* denoting a nucleus—merely single cells without a nucleus. Minimal by conventional standards, yet they are stoic, formidable survivors, and gracious givers as well. Through the action of sunlight on their chlorophyll, they built carbohydrates from water and carbon dioxide, a process called photosynthesis.

Photosynthesis not only made it possible for prokaryotes to survive without oxygen; it also added oxygen gas to earth's atmosphere. Atmospheric oxygen made feasible the evolution of more complex forms of life. Their forerunner, the eukaryotes, emerged two billion years later—single cells still, but having a nucleus containing chromosomes with genetic material. Reproducing themselves by simple division, eukaryotes remain alive in their progeny, destined never to die by natural causes. In the absence of injury, the eukaryotes are immortal. Bacteria and amoeba are members of this immortal fraternity. Mortal Homo sapiens: take note, and bow to the tiny and the minute.

1. New York: The Viking Press, 1974, p. 96.

Up to this point, life on earth was solely for the little, the uniform, the symmetrical. All were alike. All were immortal. No varieties, no creatures that fly, creep, walk, or talk. No art, no science, no poetry; no flutists, no philosophers, no prophets. No death. And no sex either. For the creation of complex, sophisticated organisms, something more than simple cellular division had to originate. By its very nature, life must continue to evolve. Answering the call, nature invented sex.

With sex on board, earth for the first time experienced an intriguing mosaic—turbulent, boisterous, and impetuous: the dawning of desire, love, lust, incest, matrimony, adultery, with the inevitability of decay, aging and death. Driven by a force mysterious, potent and compelling, chromosomes began pairing together in sexual reproduction, giving evolution its tremendous, miraculous boost. For the last 1 billion years, earth has enbraced birth and death. Going hand in hand, the two have become eternal, inseparable, compatible and interdependent. One cannot exist without the other—a fascinating coexistence of so-called absolute opposites in a faithful cycle, its revolutions constantly evoking cheer and sorrow, with some justification for both the cheer and the sorrow. (I say *justification*, not *validation*, and deliberately so.)

Certain fishes and reptiles are exempt from the mandate of eventual death; in the absence of injury, they can go on living forever. Another notable exception: some creatures are spared the rigors and ecstasy of copulation and male fertilization. Through a process known as parthogenesis they can produce a complete offspring without sexual encounters. Among those so deprived or privileged are some plants and certain invertebrate animals such as ants, bees, and ticks; but they are subject to aging and dying.

Reflecting on my own condition: I cannot escape the conclusion that my birth causes my death, so that my death will be a direct result of my birth. I also realize that I have started dying the moment I was born. To this tune I will continue dancing while my time clock keeps on ticking. I won't allow fear of death to strangle my life. Death is not foreign to me. So why hide, why panic, why lament? In and all over me, at this moment, many cells are dying while many others are being born. Some other will survive till the end of my road. I am a wandering Trimurti, a body with three heads: Brahma is creating, Shiva is destroying, while Vishnu is preserving. Me? I drink to life.

Ananda, Gautama Buddha's favorite disciple, on learning of the master's approaching death, was overcome with tears. Ananda's tears, as faithful and touching as they were, nevertheless came to be considered by the Arhats (the adepts) as a sign of his spiritual immaturity. Believing in the Law of Impermanence, even the passing of the Buddha was not to perturb them. They were schooled in the "Gatha of Impermanence":

> All composite things are impermanent,
> They are subject to birth and death;
> Put an end to birth and death,
> And there is blissful tranquility.[2]

In the spirit of the third and fourth verses, Gautama Buddha is said to have been willing to sacrifice his own life. Therefore this gatha is also frequently called the "Gatha of Sacrifice." Warriors of total freedom "are such masters of awareness, stalking, and intent that they are not caught by death, like the rest of mortal men, but choose the moment and the way of their departure from this world."[3] Often they make known the impending event by way of symbolic gestures and statements subtle or manifest, meant to transmit a well-guarded secret or proclaim concluding maxims of the sacred covenant.

In his last ceremony, Gautama Buddha affectionately offered

---

2. D. T. Suzuki, *Manual of Zen Buddhism* (New York: Grove Press, 1982), p. 15.

3. Carlos Castaneda, *The Fire from Within* (New York: Simon and Schuster, 1984), p. 13.

a lotus flower to his favorite disciple. Jesus gathered his disciples for the last supper and lovingly spoke of his impending betrayal by one of them and crucifixion. On his last pilgrimage to Mecca, Muhammad, the prophet of Islam, endearingly addressed the faithful in a farewell speech, its eloquence and high spiritual essence still alive and guiding millions of Muslims after 13 eventful centuries. Bodhidharma and Hui-neng, the first and sixth patriarchs of Zen, passed on their last testimonies to the disciples assembled around them. Hui-neng declared: "When mental activity begins, things come into being; when mental activity ceases, they too cease to exist. In parting from you, let me leave you with a stanza entitled, 'The Real Buddha of the Essence of Mind.' " Here are some of its verses of wisdom:

I hereby leave to posterity the teaching of the Sudden School[4]
For the salvation of all sentient beings who care to practice it.
Hear me, ye future disciples!
Your time will have been badly wasted if you neglect to put this teaching into practice.

Then he uttered another stanza of four lines. Having done that, he sat reverently until the third watch of the night. Then he said abruptly to his disciples, "I am going now," and in a sudden passed away.[5]

The idea of death and its inevitability ought to be a powerful incentive for living. In *A Separate Reality*, Carlos Castaneda relates what the master don Juan told him when this matter surfaced in one of their dialogues:

4. I.e. the sudden dawning of enlightenment. Though the experience is sudden, the preparation for it is often gradual and long.
5. From the Sutra of Hui-neng, trans. Wong Mou-Lam (Boulder, Co.: Shambhala Publications, 1969), p. 34.

Only the idea of death makes a man sufficiently detached so he can't deny himself anything. A man of that sort, however, does not crave, for he has acquired a silent lust for life. He knows his death is stalking him and won't give him time to cling to anything, so he tries, without craving, all of everything.

The message, then, is: let us all live life while we have it. Why waste it? The real tragedy isn't death but *what goes dead in us* while we are still alive: the desire to live; the joy of being alive; the delight in simple things; kindness; initiative; intuition; tenderness; empathy; enthusiasm; good taste; love. "What is agony of the spirit? To advance toward death without seizing hold of the Water of Life."[6]

Afterlife! What about it? Here, your guess is as good as mine. We should not contest or quarrel. The wayfarers have not returned, so let's keep an open mind. Hand me an afterlife and I'll take it! My experience in this life—modest and ambiguous by my own reckoning—will, I presume, pass on to another life. With such a lofty proposition not completely refutable at this time, let us pay attention! The wheel of life is always spinning; therefore we should feel more, see better, experience the unending mysteries, plow and experiment without regret, fear, or sense of guilt, calmly contemplating the real meaning and true nature of things. Certainly, whatever comes after will be shaped, at least in part, by what is happening right now.

If afterlife is but a dream, an imagined paradise or hell, and this life is all we have got, the conclusion is pretty obvious: let us at once concentrate. There is a whole lot of life around, all around, at all times—effervescent, vivacious, and thrilling, with much more bounty than you and I can ever afford to take. Lift the blinders and open your being, your whole being, all the way. The world is being created—*now*.

6. William C. Chittick, *The Sufi Path of Love: The Spiritual Teaching of Rumi* (Albany, N.Y.: State University of New York Press, 1983), p. 213.

Aging: How to Cope with It

With mirth and laughter let old age come.
—William Shakespeare

FROM DUSK TO DARK, THE IMAGOES SWARM IN A tragic mating dance—frantic, obsessed, doomed. Death follows. All beginning, all ending, in one day; climactic, hectic, quick. And the fugitive mayfly keeps on dancing, not knowing—I assume—that some other insects may live for 30 years; certain beetles do. Man's old friend and confidant, his ancient messenger and all-time trusted letter-carrier, the pigeon, may live for 35 years. Gregarious, always proposing and sweethearting, this good-natured bird outlives most others. In happy feathers and flamboyant color the canary sings for over 20 years. Even in a cage, the well-bred pet goes on trilling, oblivious of its confinement, accepting—perhaps, protesting! The nightingale, ghostwriter of rich melodies, co-author of innumerable joyous and heart-rending verses, confessor and consoler of forlorn lovers, and traveling companion of the solitary poet. Be it day, be it night, the nightingale sings; still, in a matter of three and a half years, the passionate cantor must fall silent.

A giant tortoise may become 177 years old, and a toothless, slow box turtle can go 123 years, far outliving its water congener, which can only make it to 7. Goats (naughty—some like them, some don't—versatile, though): billie grows a wise beard; nanny produces low-fat, easily digestible milk; angoras and cashmeres make soft fluffy wool; all within a lifespan of 18 years. Of men and mice, for better or worse, the former may kick about for 115 years; the latter for only 3. Of elephants and horses, 57 and 62 years seem to be the recorded upper limit.

On to the plant kingdom—a fascinating, vast domain, often unappreciated and rarely well understood. Take a good look at the crisp meadows at dawn: among fragrant daffodills, overnight mushroom caps rise—fresh, misty, and plump; still, in a few days the delicate, pretty things wither away, while in the White Mountains of California ancient Bristlecone pines stand patient and aloof, witnessing 4700 calendar years—secretive, assertive, with a regal air of imperial continuity.

Aging is the hallmark of individuality. Organisms merging in colonial forms without a separate existence do not age. Individual entities that we are, we cannot escape the phenomenon of aging, yet we can delay its mandated arrival, slow its progress, and with it keep a graceful company. While the human organism as a whole is mortal, yet under exceptional circumstances, a colony of human cells may live seemingly forever. Henrietta Lacks, a young black woman, died of cervical cancer on October 4, 1951. A few cells taken from her fatal growth miraculously continue to thrive to this day in a laboratory dish at Johns Hopkins Hospital School of Medicine in Baltimore. Further, the vigorous "He-La" cells, named after *Henrietta Lacks*, managed to find their way to scientific laboratories worldwide, where they dwell, live, and multiply 40 + years after Henrietta died.

Old age doesn't have to be lonesome and grim. "This is the happiest time of my life," Beatrice Woods cheerfully mused; "I know I am 90 because people tell me." She enthusiastically added: "I am never bored."[1] A renowned ceramics artist, Beatrice lives and still works at Ojai, California; she is past her middle 90s. Old age should never be conceived of as a heavy burden or a divine curse, something hard to endure. Instead: a favor. Indeed, it is. "Never resent growing old; think of the millions who are denied the privilege!" chimed in Maurice Chevalier, ever witty, lovable, and suave—the debonair legend of musical comedy who gave us *Can-Can*, *Gigi*, and *Fanny*, masterpieces among other memorable films of his. Old age does

1. From an interview with Connie Goldman, a series of conversations on the subjects of aging and creativity. Audio Production Department, University of Wisconsin–Extension, Madison, Wisconsin.

not mean quit and retire. Victor Hugo once said, "I am now 74 and I am beginning my career."

With better hygiene and improved medical care, more and more humans live longer and longer. At the beginning of the twentieth century, life expectancy in the U.S.A. was only 47 years. In 1985 it reached 71 for men and exceeded 78 for women; yet the upper limit of longevity, interestingly enough, has not changed since the time of the ancient Egyptian Pharaohs, remaining approximately 115 years.

At this time more than 24 million Americans are over age 65. Contrary to popular notions, the vast majority enjoy good health. The idea that "old age" is a disease in itself is untrue—a despicable myth refuted by the facts. It is a misleading and harmful metaphor that once and for all must be denounced and laid to rest. Deterioration of the mind known as dementia is not a constant comrade of the aged. Alzheimer's disease, much dreaded by the elderly, their families, and friends, afflicts no more than 5 percent over 65 and 18 percent above 85. To improve the outlook even further: 15 to 30 percent of those diagnosed as having Alzheimer's have dementia caused by malnutrition, infection, head injury, or some other treatable condition.

Depression and schizophrenia are much more widespread than Alzheimer's disease; and with appropriate treatment, both are curable or, at the very least, controllable. Statements like Montaigne's "Our mind grows constipated and sluggish as it grows old" are meritless and false. They do injustice to the elderly, tarnishing their image, limiting their potential, and diminishing their self-esteem. Such should be mentioned only to be condemned.

The wise prepare early on for aging. Waiting until one gets in there, then fighting and resisting, or bowing and accepting, is unwise. Mysterious as it is, the process of aging is influenced by five conditions: one's genetic makeup; one's attitude; environment; physical activity; and nutrition. All but one are to a great extent subject to our control. Certainly we can work on them to a decisive advantage.

The genetic blueprint for life is still obscure, though not for long. Researchers have already mapped more than 1000 individual genes—a modest fraction of the 50,000 to 100,000 determining a person's makeup; but scientists realistically foresee a complete map of human genes by the year 2000. A specific gene determining or regulating the speed of aging has not yet been conclusively identified. If one is pinpointed—and reliable clues indicate that this possibility is indeed valid—the scope of what lies ahead in terms of gene therapy is awesome and thrilling. Extending the lifespan and improving the human stock are not anymore the impossible dream they once were. They may happen. I dare say, they will. Good?—or bad? Good *and* bad? Can't tell for sure. "It all depends!"

The Influence of One's Attitude
on Aging

ONE'S OWN ATTITUDE CAN MAKE A DIFFERENCE—AN appreciable one. As years and birthdays pile up, we tend to give up things, duties and hobbies alike. Doing so, we—knowingly or unknowingly—become sluggish, bored, and boring, eventually turning pathetic and apathetic, thus helplessly embracing senility and infirmity. Still busy painting at 95, Zhu Quizhan, one of four living monarchs of Chinese painting, gleefully vowed, "I will never stop painting." Of bamboo, his favorite subject, he said, "It never breaks and it goes its own way. That is how I see myself." Pleading never to stop painting, never to break, Zhu did just that. His most recent calligraphic brushworks and color concepts did not lose earlier brilliance or zeal, remaining vivacious and irresistibly engaging.

Albert Schweitzer continued to work in Lambaréné, western Gabon, until his death in 1965 at age 90. Natives of Lambaréné were utterly helpless and desperately ill. Experiencing their wretchedness and great misfortune, Schweitzer could not walk away entrusting it all to the hands of almighty God or someone else. He stayed on, founded his hospital there in 1913, and made Lambaréné his home.

Unfortunately, with the outbreak of World War I in 1914, not even the shanty town was spared the wrath and disgrace of the cruel war. The living saint and his wife were taken to a prison camp. The sole accusation: being German. The shrill cries of the frail, the unbearable suffering of unweaned children, logic, common sense, or even pity—none mattered. During the infamous years of incarceration, the prisoner wrote his creed, *The Reverence for Life*. Returning to Lambaréné in 1924, he resumed his volunteer work, which kept him very busy for 51 more years. For the love of Albert and in appreciation, the people of Lambaréné bestowed on him their highest honor, "Oganga of Lambaréné," meaning "fetishman working magic." The Nobel Prize came in 1953, money from which went to buy more supplies for the hospital.

In his autobiography, Albert Schweitzer wrote, "It struck me as incomprehensible that I should be allowed to lead such a happy life while I saw so many people around wrestling with care and suffering." In his heart, the saint cradles suffering and joy, embracing both: he mends and heals, all while his spirit is loving and serene. To propagate love and serenity, his own spirit must, in essence, be love and serenity. Young at 90, Albert died content. His reverence for life will live to inspire the compassionate, move the indifferent, and transform the cruel. "Everyone can have his own Lambaréné." This, one of Schweitzer's sayings, is the essence of his story.

"But there is a lot of good living after 65 if you have an interesting life," said Hulda Crooks as she approached the 14,494-foot summit of Mt. Whitney. Undaunted at 90, the Loma Linda widow successfully climbed the treacherous 11-mile trail to the high peak in August 1986—her twenty-third successful climb. Diminutive, sprightly, witty, and vegetarian, she began mountain climbing and jogging at the age of 66—generally considered time to withdraw and slumber. Not for Hulda! She walks three and a half miles every day and wanted to make at least two more ascents of Mt. Whitney. In July 1987, she made it to the lofty summit of Japan's Mt. Fuji. Why does she do it? Hulda replies, "Older people tend to feel their lives are over when they reach 65. . . . You must always have hope for the future." An exhilarating remark.

Vow never to retire, never to quit. If you are self-employed do not close your books. If Uncle Sam or the corporation takes you off active service, search high and low for a piece of work, something meaningful to do to keep your wits active and your frame energetic. If you do not need to earn your keep, volunteer, help another. So many in this world urgently need help and still hope to get it. Their hope has been deferred for so long, and we know it. All that is left for them is their freedom to hope. This is their only raft; do not let it sink. Waiting for Godot, Vladimir passionately implored Estragon, "To all mankind they were addressed, those cries for help still ringing in our ears! But at this place, at this moment of time, all mankind is us."[1]

A great many good causes are here, right here, at this moment, at this place, waiting for sponsor and support. Choose one, select any: the complex dilemma of the poor, the plight of the hungry, the tragedy of the homeless, the predicament of the missing, the spiritual humiliation and physical hurt of the battered, the deprivation of the illiterate, kids hooked on dope, adults intoxicated with alcohol, the case for animal rights, environmental pollution, acid rain, peace on earth, energy conservation, political reform. Connecting ourselves to causes beyond ourselves and past our personal needs confers on us a perpetual reason to be, a ceaseless impulse to go on, an immunity of sorts.

Memory recalls the pitiful downfall of some of our glamorous celebrities and admired role models. Having reached the summit they always dreamed and struggled to achieve, all of a sudden their inner drive came to a halt and incomprehensibly they slipped into neurotic withdrawal. Shocking and sad, witnessing those who went adrift and the others who took their own lives amidst the limelight and the glitter of gold, fame, and applause. Self-interested, notorious egocentrics, outside themselves they could behold nothing—only vast emptiness, an unfriendly terrain visited by the yellow wind of boredom and rusty repetition. The beautiful world of yesterday had turned ugly, flickering with frightening reflections and inverted images, inhabited by remote, unworthy dwarfs. No place to live. The poor soul was swallowed in its darkness and demise.

If you have a hobby, you are fortunate; keep at it. Young or old, do not let it go. If you have none, begin one. Write a novel. Life is eventful, brimming with stories to tell; narrate one.

1. Samuel Beckett, *Waiting for Godot* (New York: Grove Press, 1954), p. 51.

Compose a poem. Let your verses arrange themselves; decorum and poetic splendor will dawn by themselves. Only, be true to what moves you.

Paint a portrait of someone interesting or beloved. At first special features, style, and color may be lacking; but your sincere enthusiasm will nurture your art and cause it to grow and flourish. Sketch a scene you like; there must be many. If you cannot recall any, open your eyes or scratch your head a little. Soon you will find the missing picture book in the library of your mind. Reproduce it, bring it out.

You may turn your head away or laugh at your first amateurish product, but do not forget: defects will correct themselves as the brain and the hands get accustomed to working together and relating better to one another. The artist's reward will come; give it time, do not rush it, do not despair, do not quit.

Sculpture the beautiful and the vulnerable, carve a figurine, or run your feeling fingers into a virgin lump of clay; your eager hands will someday get it right. Photograph people, meadows, hills, birds, trees, and flowers—so much to capture and to project from the angle you think will reveal beauty at its best.

In rapt quietude, garden your back yard. Plants show their appreciation in pleasing colors, sweet fragrance, fruits and blossoms; in divine silence, watch them grow. Tilling the patient, wistful, never impassive soil is reputed to be a virtue.

On an early Sunday morning, treat your routine self to something unusual: mixing some dough, waiting for it to rise, baking it in the oven—purifying pieces of work, slighted and forgotten; yet bread has for long been revered as a symbolic staff of life, of sharing, of fraternity and modesty in eating. Have we forgotten?

Hike the parks and trails, travel the world, read about what you do not know, learn more about what you think you know, play music, dance, dance, dance. Said the muse in *My Fair Lady*, ''I could have danced all night.'' Cheers!

Somewhere, sometime along the circling roads of life, each must have longed to do something really neat, really interesting, exciting, perhaps challenging—yet for one reason or another never got to achieve it. Well, the case is not closed; on the horizon there are always second and third chances. It is never too late. Chance and opportunity are of two different kinds: one blooms from a source within, self-generated; the other is external, independent of our control. External chance and opportunity, sweet and ardently wished for by everyone, are seasonless and timeless. They follow stars unknown to us, dawning and smiling even when we least expect them, yet always favoring the prepared mind.

Self-generated chance and opportunity exist at all times, hovering around, perpetually circulating the inner sphere of our own perception, and subject to our will. It's up to us to "get with it," move on, and keep our inner spark kindled and live. We must not permit our spirit to slacken or despair. If we do, there is nothing to accuse but our own ineptitude.

Environment Counts:
Its Influence on Aging

ENVIRONMENT COUNTS. DON QUIXOTE, LOOKING about the plaza, hears figures huddled below the stairs and against the wall of the town whispering about their loneliness. He leans upon his lance and says, "When so many are lonely as seem to be lonely, it would be inexcusably selfish to be lonely alone."[1] Inexcusable.

There is no reasonable reason to be lonesome. Something begs to be done. Humanity's lonely spectacle cannot be ignored; it is bleak, it is dreary, it is selfish. To every lonely soul: don't make the error of waiting; another lonely soul may be waiting for you, and all may end up waiting, embracing their despairing loneliness. Waiting and waiting. Just waiting. Everybody waiting.

Such waiting is meaningless, senseless, humorless. It is up to us to define its meaning, purpose, and limits. When strangers meet and silence grows uneasy, one or the other has the obligation of breaking the uneasy silence. Take the initiative, let it be you, extend yourself, open the dialogue, bridge the gap. Empathy, friendship, affection, shared experiences—all frozen inside—will melt and gainfully flow out like a warm summer stream.

Many a loving and kindly emotion may bud out of the briefest chance encounter. Talk to someone. Break the artificial barrier. Bid your cranky neighbor a good day; send an ear-to-ear smile to happy children giggling and fussing while kicking the ball; warmly greet an elderly couple strolling down the sidewalk. And say hello to the cheerless, grumpy fellow cursing

---

1. Tennessee Williams, *Camino Real* (New York: New Directions, Spring 1970), p. 6.

behind you at the supermarket check-out counter; you don't need to know him beforehand, and now you will.

Lonely people of the world: *head where people are.* Don't just sit down glued to your sofas and loungers. Step out of the remote labyrinth that has cloistered you for so long! Your self-imposed seclusion will only keep you apart. Don't be bashful; *converse.* There are multiple topics of conversation less boring than the dull weather and Uncle Sam's intrusions and indiscretions. Speak of carnations; the splendors of Babylon; the late Sir Lawrence Olivier's wrath as Othello and his splendid hesitation as Hamlet; the bewildering complexity of human behavior; the haunting, compelling characters of Lawrence Durrell's *Alexandria Quartet*; the immortal monuments consecrating the banks of the Nile River; the happy and unhappy tales of the Rio Grande; the Buddha's enlightenment and compassion; the magic of lasers; romantic gondolas drifting along the canals of Venice; Troy's lost treasures; Cyrano's hopeless love for Roxanne; the land and seaborne adventures of the seagull; today's political cartoon in your local newspaper; the acrobatics, fillibusters, and meddlings of the U.S. Congress; covert government policies; the tango's erotic elegance; the heartfelt throb of jazz; and a million other subjects.

To find yours, dip your hand in the jar, pick a fortune cookie, open it. And if you prefer listening: the male crickets are chirping and a distant frog is croaking.

Stop judging others; quit calling them unfriendly, aloof, egotistic, cold. They may be merely timid, just like you. Their judgment of you may be as harsh as yours of them. In all fairness, very few human beings are all that reserved, consciously cool, genuinely suspicious, or hopelessly rude and inconsiderate. Your warm gentle touch will peel off the outer cold wrappings. The hides might be tough leather; but the core, the matter inside, is soft and tender, ever yearning to be stirred. Inside there is warm juice, and it is the vibrations of this good stuff that make us what we are. Within all of us it is one and the same. The sulky, prickly rind differs in thickness and color; but beneath, it is all the same: good stuff testifying to our innate purity and our lost but not irrecoverable innocence.

> All Adam's race are members of one frame;
> Since all, at first, from the same essence came.[2]

As we drop the cloak of indifference, we should remember and recall to the center of our daily lives two of our most benevolent allies: pets and plants—always there to help, never failing to answer our call. To the lonely who insist on being solitaire, they come to the rescue. There is always that hardy lot, stubborn, vainly deriding the selfishness and conceit of others, constantly denouncing the world, but by no means acknowledging the same faults in themselves. Clinging to their loneliness, their lives run stale; their days go sluggish; their nights are cold, long, and wearisome. Yet these disaffected souls secretly crave company and are dying for a friendly touch or a warm embrace—though never admitting it.

Without fanfare, pets and plants can quietly step in, fulfilling their needs. Companionship of pets and plants takes the chill away, imparting a measure of self-discipline and an atmosphere of liveliness that enrich the human environment. Overwhelming evidence confirms the psychologic enhancement that the elderly and lonely can gain from closely associating with pets and plants. All along, these wonderful creations have given humankind far more than they have ever received. Goodness is in their fundamental nature.

Can retirement and nursing homes be of help to the elderly? My answer is a flat *No*. Retirement homes signal resignation. No matter how plush, how roomy, how tidy, they spell dejection. The incredible boom in nursing and convalescent homes is scandalous and insane. A lack of love; fading affection— something has broken already, is breaking, or is going to break.

2. Sheikh M. Sadi, *The Rose Garden*, trans. E. B. Eastwick (London: The Octagon Press, 1979), p. 38. A contemporary of Jalal al-Din Rumi, Sadi was called the "Nightingale of a Thousand Songs."

It is all a byproduct of the dissolution of the family's cohesive structure by the lure of economic gain, the powerful magnet of upward mobility, the idleness of convenience, the misinterpreted call for personal freedom, the imagined needs, and the expediency of a society that prefers satiety to satisfaction; trimming, garnish, and exotic dressing to natural wholesomeness; bigness to beauty; sedation to calm; electronic buzz and flicker to cozy concord with fellow creatures; speed to efficiency; waste to conservation; and good looks to experience.

Let the social elite and contemporary role models have all that nonsense; let them hoard all the pretty gadgets. Let the neophytes, the pseudosociologists, the constipated executives, the flat-headed short-sighted futurists preach the new religion. Let them all snort, purse their lips, and turn their noses up. However, they cannot disguise a fundamental fact: the family is society's building block, indeed its nucleus. Fractured or strained, the entire structure collapses on its inhabitants. And it is a silent, invisible breakdown—no smoke, no ashes, no stink; not even the audible thunder-clap of a modest explosion.

Our five senses may not sense the momentous shatter, but see what happens: alienation, hard drugs, alcohol, stress, depression, and crime consuming the young, with abandonment and abuse befalling the old. A costly enterprise for which a quick fix is unforeseen unless we have the courage and vision to make a turn in the right direction.

Forgive me for activating the alarm; I am merely reporting what I see.

Exercise: Its Effect on Aging

EXERCISE IS NOT ALIEN TO THE HUMAN BODY; IT IS most natural. We are not designed to be stiff or stationary. Why do we have 600 muscles which, pulled in one direction, could lift 25 tons? Our skeleton has 206 bones perfectly connected together by smooth, movable joints—to what end? More than half of those 206 bones are in our hands and feet; there must be a good reason. Our tireless heart muscle pumps more than five quarts of blood every minute, 2000 gallons a day—for whom? for what? Our bones are hardy; one cubic inch can withstand a two-ton force. Wherefore?

Begun in childhood and continued throughout life, physical exercise is most helpful. It upgrades the mechanical efficiency and endurance level of the heart. By lowering the blood pressure, exercise can help prevent or lessen hardening of our blood vessels, a disease known as atherosclerosis (a form of arteriosclerosis). Arteriosclerosis is the primary cause of heart attacks and strokes. These two afflictions take a high toll, claiming the lives of 800,000 Americans annually in addition to disabling many more.

Diabetes mellitus is a disease with many victims that spawns serious complications ruining our kidneys, eyes, and blood vessels, compromising our ability to heal even minor cuts or bruises and undermining our natural immunity, thus making us susceptible to a host of infections. Fortunately, its severity can to a certain degree be controlled, its onset possibly delayed, and, in some instances, the disease itself even altogether prevented—by exercise. While exercising, muscles burn calories, putting insulin to work. Insulin is a potent hormone secreted by the pancreas; it performs multiple functions, the foremost of which is regulation of the blood-sugar level. If this function is slightly deranged or minimally interfered with, diabetes develops and progresses.

Arthritis is a crippling, painful disease that torments the old and the young and for which there is no effective remedy in most cases. Judicious motion of different parts of the body can be crucial in bringing relief or enhancing the possibility of a cure or a long remission. Inactivity causes bone resorption, a condition known as osteoporosis. The once sturdy skeleton turns porous and brittle—a setback for the most part preventable by exercise. With tougher bones, smoother joints, and well-conditioned pliable musculature, accidental injury harms us less. Agile and fit, we are less likely to loose footing; and if we do take a spill, we are the more apt to bounce back, escaping bone fractures and joint dislocations. And in the event of a break or derangement, the damage is more often contained and heals faster. Such are the benefits of exercise.

Exercise also elevates mood and restores stamina. It gives a substantial boost to the immune system—our natural defense mechanism against not only infections but also against a potential and most dreaded enemy: cancer. Almost miraculously, our body can sense the early budding of cancer or malignancy in any of its parts. Different tissues and organs are patrolled by a sophisticated surveillance system constantly cruising our territories, everywhere intercepting and killing any cell that looks abnormal or behaves accordingly.

Cancer cells are aberrant and have distinctive features under the microscope. Besides being larger in size, they multiply faster and invade neighboring organs. The hyperactive cells may reach remote sites such as the liver, brain, bones or lungs by way of the blood stream and lymphatic network. They do not obey any of the body's regulatory mechanisms the way normal cells do, so they are described as autonomous.

A healthy immune system is alert; it recognizes and destroys the unruly cells. Throughout life, apparently, cancer cells keep sprouting. But for a vigilant immune system, the ''autonomous'' ones would have it their way, growing up to be avid tumors that would literally eat us up to ultimate extinction.

Individuals who are depressed, pessimistic, cynical, with a negative outlook, sluggish physique, and an attitude of giving up suffer higher cancer rates and are commonly stricken with greater ferocity. They are the same kind of people who are less likely to follow discipline, more apt to indulge and to pick up bad habits such as smoking, drinking, and overeating. Besides, their compliance with prevention or treatment protocols is suboptimal to nil. The grim disease consumes them quicker.

On the contrary, those with cheerful disposition, optimistic mental attitude, healthy habits, and active physique are afflicted with cancer less often. Struck, they stand a better chance of conquering the disease and surviving the adversity—or, at the very least, of subduing its intensity and of suffering less.

Physical exercise knows no age limit. The important element is to start early on; but if one misses this early calling, still, "better late than never." For the late newcomers—those 40 and above—first, consult your physician. In particular, the condition of the heart must be checked out. Be careful; go slow and be brief to begin with. Add more exercise time and speed very gradually as you go along, week after week, rather than daily. Perform regularly—preferably no less than four times a week. Continue past age 60, 70, 80, or even 90.

As we've already observed, at 90, Hulda Crooks climbed Mt. Whitney's 14,494-foot peak. The following year she made it to the summit of Mt. Fuji even though she began this not-so-easy hobby at 66. I saw Fred Astaire past 85—princely, evergreen, erect, and pliant like a Norfolk Island pine, infallibly graceful. From childhood on, I have been a loyal fan of Fred Astaire. *Top Hat, Funny Face, Daddy Longlegs, Shall We Dance*, and other of his hits meant to me more—far more—than memorable entertainment. The whole thing was a way of life, a self-renewing melody, its verses and rhymes never to end. Caught in Astaire's magic, I recall intimating to myself time after time, "Boy, one day you will grow old like everyone else; let it be Astaire's way!" My heart still beats the Astaire theme, and, I am overjoyed.

Among the elderly, I witness the stout and the slim; the sluggish and the brisk; huffing, puffing cranks, and others content and at ease; some fretful and rude, some witty and sweet. I realize that each has a right to his or her own way. I admit that circumstance can be mean and overpowering. But for years I have been monitoring the human condition. From what I have seen, it isn't all circumstance and predestination, nor is it all freedom of choice and options of convenience. I see it as a perpetual interplay, a dynamic mix of both—at times random, at times orderly. While I cannot choose all my dice, still, am I not the one doing the throwing? This must have something to do with what the spots on the upturned faces total and with the outcome of the game. Maybe exercise, style, and enthusiasm aren't enough to transform an ugly duckling into a swan, but surely they can make the duck a better duck! Doing our best with what was handed to us, we shall travel our road with a smaller burden and fewer pains.

Nutrition and Aging

THE WORD "DIET" DERIVES FROM THE LATIN AND Greek, meaning "manner of life." Our way of life seems to have gone astray. Our sweet/fat tooth is giving us plenty of grief. Over the past 100 years or so, our unrestrained taste for fat and sugar has been notoriously exploited by the food industry. Toward this end, livestock selective-breeding methods are being employed, methods that are heartless, detestable, and scandalous. Adding cruelty to obscenity, newer feeding practices have come along, gruesome and ghastly, such as "finishing" cattle at feed lots with energy-enriched corn and grain.

What comes of all this mischief? The modest "lean" beef has become "well-marbled," tender, and juicy. Believe it or not, your "choice" sirloin cut draws 84 percent of its calories from fat and as little as 16 percent from protein. Amazing! But true. Contrariwise, the meat from wild animals that our ancestors ate derived 82 percent of its calories from protein and only 18 percent from fat (55 percent of which is polyunsaturated). The meat sold in your friendly supermarket has 5 percent or less polyunsaturated fat. We've come a long way! In which direction, though?

Looking around, we see street corners littered with shopping centers, themselves littered with fast-food franchises serving french fries that have more than 80 times the fat that baked potatoes have. The sumptuous menu features even more delights: sour cream; an assortment of exotic salad dressings; butter; supersweet pastries; prepared mixes; soft drinks; richly flavored shakes; and don't forget: ice cream in all flavors and colors. All soaked with fat and inundated with sugar. Our children eagerly gulp down these sensuous treats, happily—and as though in a stupor—getting used to the rewarding, mellow taste of fat and the enticing sweetness of sugar. For the rest of their lives, this can be what they'll crave and ask for. Complex carbohydrates such as baked potatoes, steamed rice, plain bread are uninteresting items; dry, flavorless, tasteless. Their austere nature must be improved, served buttered or fried, sprinkled with sugar or drenched in syrup. That will do the trick. Enjoy! Enjoy! Fiber (as in bran and vegetables) is for the rabbits.

From all that we know, taste is a dictate of habit. I, for one, will not strip a freshly baked potato of its heavenly taste by adding butter or sour cream, nor stifle the aroma and wholesome savor of freshly baked bread with garnish or margarine. A great many vegetables fresh or steamed have innate flavor, a subtle natural fragrance. The frying pan steals away this relish. Conditioned, we reflexly reach for the sweet, the salt and the grease, thus doing away with the original distinctive tastes of what we eat.

Without these customary additions, we might even choke: with chewing and mastication practically forgotten, a hardy food item has no chance to soften; a dry article remains arid. Our own saliva, not mayonnaise, or butter, is the natural lubricant of food, ensuring smooth transit down our delicate esophagus. Saliva's enzymes are meant to initiate the digestion of nutrients, facilitating the subsequent work of the stomach.

Ingredients now lacking in our meals were plentiful in our forefathers' diet. Fossilized bones prove that these people were strongly built. The Cro-Magnons, who inhabited Europe between 35,000 and 10,000 years ago, were taller than today's Americans. In 1984 came the amazing discovery of a nearly complete fossilized skeleton of Homo erectus—a more distant ancestor of ours. It clearly shows that 1.6 million years ago people equaled us in height. Our ancestors were not the dwarfs and midgets we think they were. True, many of them died young, but this was mostly due to infection and injury, both of which we can control to a substantial degree. Their elders rarely suffered heart attacks, hypertension, stroke, obesity, diabetes, and cancer—collectively dubbed ''diseases of civilization.'' Contemporary hunter-gatherers have a health profile comparable to that of our forbears. This is no invitation to go hunting or to support the National Rifle Association. No. Prudently selecting the best from our ancestors' lifestyle and from our own as well, we are bound to live longer and become healthier.

We are not ready for our contemporary "feast" yet! So far, our metabolic pathways have not made the adjustment necessary to handle the new, excessive dietary supply of fat—in particular, saturated fat—and refined sugars in a safe, efficient manner. It takes time; thousands of years, millions perhaps. The wheel of biologic adaptation turns slowly, very slowly. We are running ahead of the wheel, way ahead. We diverged from the chimpanzee nearly seven million years ago; still, surprisingly, our genes and theirs differ by a mere 1.5 percent. At this time, our metabolic pathways have not yet learned how to cope with much of the stuff we eat and drink. Their failure is manifested as "diseases of civilization."

Increase in the total amount of dietary fat renders us more susceptible to cancers of the breast, prostate, uterus, pancreas, and colon. Chinese women living in Taiwan consume small amounts of fat; their estrogen hormone levels are relatively low, and so is their incidence of breast cancer. In Honolulu, Chinese American women eat fat in moderate proportions, have higher estrogen levels, and a moderately high incidence of breast cancer. As Bostonians do, Chinese American women living in Boston do: helping themselves to excess fat, they have high estrogen levels, and the incidence of breast cancer among them matches that of white American women—high. Looking at prostatic cancer, similar trends are noted. Black American men eat a rich fat diet, have higher testosterone levels, and suffer more prostatic cancer than black Nigerian men do.

As if this weren't enough, here is some more: A high fat intake stimulates the liver to secrete more bile. Bacteria normally inhabiting the colon break bile acids into a number of chemical compounds believed to be carcinogenic. In their newly earned material affluence, many Japanese are adding more and more fat to their diet and adding more and more cancers to their colons. Dietary fiber in sufficient amounts stimulates bowel movement, thereby preventing constipation and reducing the colon's bacterial count and colonic cancer as well. Several well-controlled epidemiologic studies have confirmed this favorable finding. Finland's low rate of colon cancer has been linked to eating baked foods and cereals made from whole grains. Over the past three decades, cancer death rates have increased steadily. According to the National Cancer Institute, too much fat and too little fiber account for one-third of all cancer.

Dietary fat has three varieties: saturated, polyunsaturated, and monounsaturated. The indispensable essential fatty acids are all polyunsaturated. Our body cannot make them, therefore our diet must supply them. Certain vital components of our cellular structure and some necessary hormones cannot be synthesized in the absence of these fatty acids. Furthermore, polyunsaturated (and possibly monounsaturated) fats lower blood cholesterol levels, while saturated fats raise those levels. High blood cholesterol contributes to hardening of the arteries (arteriosclerosis) and hence to coronary heart disease. Compared to Americans, Japanese and many Third World peoples consume less fat, but with proportionately more of the polyunsaturated variety in what fat they do eat. They suffer fewer heart attacks than Americans.

The typical American diet provides 40–50 percent calories from fat, two-thirds of which is saturated. Outrageous. Ideally, only 20–25 percent of the daily calories ought to come from fat, with preference for the polyunsaturated (as in olive oil and fish oils). This diet will lower high blood cholesterol. Lest all seem rosy and secure, a note of caution: too much of *any* dietetic ingredient, even an apparently innocent one, can harm. There is a suspicion that excess polyunsaturated fats may increase our risk of getting cancer. Moderation and temperance are the key; they pay off.

At this point, let's note that the habit of smoking merits outright condemnation. Suicidal. Homicidal, it harms others who breathe while you smoke. It predisposes human lungs to cancer, now the number-one killer among all cancers afflicting both sexes. The National Cancer Institute estimates that tobacco is responsible for 30 percent of cancers. It also causes emphysema, a progressively destructive lung disease that literally takes the breath away. Cancer of the urinary bladder and esophagus are more frequent in smokers. Our tender hearts and pliable blood vessels cannot stand the stuff that does them substantial injury. Smokers have comparatively much higher rates of heart attacks and major blood circulation problems in different parts of the body. Quit. Quit. Nonsmokers, do not stay near those who smoke. They pollute the air you will soon be inhaling, charging it with carcinogens that will harm you as well.

The second edition of *Nutrition and Your Health: Directory Guidelines for Americans* was released in 1985 as *Home and Garden Bulletin No. 232*. The revised diet guidelines are:

Eat a variety of foods.

Maintain desirable weight.

Avoid too much fat, saturated fat, and cholesterol.

Eat foods with adequate starch and fiber.

Avoid too much sugar.

Avoid too much sodium.

If you drink alcoholic beverages, do so in moderation.

In this context, it is timely to have a brief, clear look at alcohol. Alcohol is not a drink; it is a drug—plain and simple. Labeling alcohol as a drink and believing it is naive and misleading, serving only to domesticate a powerful chemical, promoting it as an article of hospitality, a toast for all occasions and a friend of the lonesome and the burned-out. The drug plays havoc with our indispensable liver and inflicts substantial damage on the stomach, esophagus, and pancreas. Several acute and chronic catastrophic illnesses may develop as a direct result. Our heart is not spared the wrath; its vital muscle fibers are shot down by alcohol. Bit by bit, the heart's ability to pump and keep blood circulating dwindles down—a fatal condition known as cardiomyopathy. Fatal as it is, cardiomyopathy has very few early warning signals, sneaking in and usually diagnosed when it is too late to help its unfortunate victim. And our traffic toll, high and grim, is directly caused by alcohol in over 50 percent of instances.

As if all these misfortunes were not sufficient to fill the cup of sorrow, here is another: alcohol assaults our higher brain centers, inducing a state of mind inclined to domestic violence—a growing menace threatening our civility and lives. Society's complacency with alcohol is groundless, senseless, and hypocritical. It is high time to be honest about it, face facts, and include alcohol in all our antidrug campaigns.

Back to *Nutrition and Your Health*: relative to fat and cholesterol, the following recommendations ought to guide food selection:

Choose lean meat, fish, and poultry.

Use skim or low-fat milk and meat products.

Moderate the use of egg yolk and organ meats.

Limit intake of fats and oils, especially those high in saturated fat and foods containing palm and coconut oils.

Trim fat off meat.

Broil, bake, or boil rather than fry.

Moderate the use of foods that contain fat, such as breaded and deep-fried foods.

Read labels carefully to determine both amount and type of fat present in food.[1]

A balanced diet with a variety of foods along these guidelines supplies vitamins and minerals; however, I can't quarrel with anyone taking supplements of one or both, since I personally do.

1. *Yearbook of Science and the Future* (Encyclopedia Britannica, Inc., 1987), p. 396.

Eating: Moral Issues of Relevance—with a Word on the Health, Social, and Ecologic Problems Linked to a Meat-Centered Diet

STOPPING FOR REFLECTION: EATING POSES A MORAL dilemma of sorts. I see the bird eating the worm and devouring the grain, the spider entangling and feasting on the fly, the lizard gulping the moth, the cat chasing and ravenously eating the mouse, big fish feeding on small fish, and certain plants attracting and trapping insects. I see you and me consuming animals and plants to satisfy hunger or satiate appetite. A mutual eating society, isn't it? As though our very survival couldn't survive without terminating another's survival. Painfully true! In my humble opinion: this is the "Universal Sin"—a mandate of necessity! Or so it seems.

Obligatory and innate; then *does* it constitute a sin? If it qualifies as one: is it pardonable? Can we atone and make up for it? Is there an alternative? Is there a way out of this transgression short of inanition and death? Starving one's self to death is a prima facie act of suicide. We're told that suicide is a form of homicide, strictly forbidden, a sin—ungodly, unpardonable.

At every crossroad, the human conscience is being tested and challenged. The crowd—caring less—looks the other way, bypassing the burden of personal responsibility. Certain religions command the faithful to abstain from what is meat. Distressed by animals' suffering and the guilt of taking their lives, many opt for vegetarianism. Some ethicists reach the same decision through philosophical thinking and diligent soul-searching. The question still remains: will vegetarianism wipe the slate clean? Will it absolve mankind of the guilt of sacrificing other lives for the sake of its own survival?

Hindu scientists convincingly proved that plants feel the injury of mutilation and do suffer. Rooted in the soil, plants

134

cannot run away. Their cry goes silent; so do ultrasound, undertones, and many whispers—inaudible by our ears. Their delicate quiver remains unseen, like ultraviolet light, infrared rays, and the fundamental movement within every atom. Jagadis C. Bose[1] noted the parallels between animal and plant tissues. Using very sensitive, automatic instruments, Bose recorded extremely small movements interpreted as apparent feeling of injury in plants. Hurt, they tremble. "This is the reason why we must talk to plants we are about to kill and apologize for hurting them; the same thing must be done with the animals we are going to hunt."[2]

At this juncture certain research data on the health, social, and ecologic problems linked to a meat-centered diet ought to be told.[3]

World Hunger

Number of humans who will starve to death
this year: 60,000,000
Number of humans who could be adequately fed by
grain saved if Americans reduced their intake of
meat by 10%: 60,000,000
Pounds of grain and soybeans needed to produce
1 pound of feedlot beef: 16
Percentage of corn grown in United States eaten by
human beings: 20
Percentage of corn grown in United States eaten by
livestock: 80
Pounds of potato that can be grown on 1 acre of land: 2000
Pounds of beef that can be produced on 1 acre of land: 165

1. Jagadis C. Bose, *The Nervous Mechanism of Plants* (New York: Longmans, Green and Co., 1926).
2. Carlos Castaneda, *A Separate Reality* (New York: Pocket Books, 1971), p. 226.
3. The following excerpts are from John Robbins, *Diet for a New America* (Walpole, N.H.: Stillpoint Publishing, 1987).

Health Care

Most common cause of death in U.S.: heart attack
Risk of death from heart attack by average
American man: 50%
Risk of heart attack by average American
pure vegetarian man: 4%
Increased risk of breast cancer for women who
eat meat daily compared to pure vegetarian women:
5 times higher
Increased risk of prostate cancer for men who consume
meat and dairy products compared to pure vegetarian men:
3.6 times higher
Increased risk of colon cancer for people who eat meat
and dairy products as compared to pure vegetarians:
10 times higher

Natural Resources: Consumption and Pollution

More than half the water consumed in the U.S. is for:
livestock production
Water needed to produce 1 pound of wheat: 25 gallons
Water needed to produce 1 pound of meat: 2500 gallons
Percentage of water pollution due to organic waste from
U.S. Humans: 10
Percentage of water pollution due to organic waste from
U.S. livestock: 90

Consumption of Pesticides

Source of pesticide residues in the U.S. diet:
meat—55%; dairy products—23%; vegetables—6%;
fruits—4%; grains—1%
Percentage of male college students sterile in 1950: 0.5
Percentage of male college students sterile in 1978: 25

Principal reason for sterility and sperm count reduction
in U.S. males: pesticide residues
Percentage of U.S. mother's milk containing dangerous
levels of DDT: 99

Rain Forest and Species Survival

Driving force behind the (6 acre/minute) destruction of the
life-supporting, oxygen-producing Central American
rainforests: creation of grazing land to grow beef for export
Current rate of species extinction due to destruction of
Central American rainforests and related habitants: 1000/year
Amount of trees spared per year by each individual who
switches to a pure vegetarian diet: 1 acre

Political Tensions

Barrels of oil imported daily by U.S.: 6,800,000
Principal reason for U.S. military intervention in
Persian Gulf: dependence on foreign oil
Amount of imported oil U.S. needs to meet present demand
if 10% of population became fully vegetarian: none

For our very existence, bodily nutrition is, of course, imperative. No matter which way we choose to look at it, our existence is not a free enterprise, it is not self-sustaining; it subsists at a tremendous expense: that of other lives. Maintained at a dreadfully high cost, our life must have a purpose, a meaning, some value, a certain promise. Wouldn't it be a shame and a pity to waste it? Certainly ungrateful and unworthy to use it to harm, diminish, or destroy one's own self or others. In life's covenant, "others" reads: *humans, animals, plants,* and *environment.* In the well-guarded covenant, all are included as one. Such a wasteful destructive course of action stares human-kind right in the face as cowardly and abominable. A mortal sin. Live, let live; love, let love; gain, let gain; heal, let heal; wander, let wander; be free, let be free; worship, let worship. Our personal pursuit of happiness will be consummated only by giving happiness to others.

Every action has a reaction that bounces back on the doer. Pain and grief repay pain and grief; kindness and caring return as kindness and caring. The form of the rendering might differ, but in effect and essence it matches the original act that triggered it in the first place. The happy tune is ours, if we play it. This is the way to make amends and expiate for the sin of taking other lives to nurture our own. It is a "Deed of Trust." Without our carrying our part, the Universal Sin will not wash out, will stick to us, tarnishing our psyche and clouding our intellect.

The "mark of Cain" is acquired, individual, delible, curable. Human wrongdoings ever yearn to be cleared. If this basic understanding is affirmed by realization and crowned by fulfilling our obligation in the "Deed of Trust," the habit of eating is then purified of its moral repercussions. Living to eat is immoral and wasteful. It is unkind, unhealthy, ultimately self-destructive.

Laying no claim to originality, and without condescending or patronizing, I'd like to share with you some practical guidelines. Following them, I found solution to several of my own serious trepidations about eating. A measure of comfort and internal serenity followed, with better digestion as well.

1. For the sake of our senses of taste and smell, food ought to be palatable and agreeable; this helps its digestion. Modest, yes; exquisite and consummate, no; otherwise it is likely to stimulate desire for more and may unleash and open up appetite, thereby inviting gluttony. Gluttony perverts the human lot, corrupting body and spirit. Every religion and moral creed has opposed gluttony.

2. "Eat only when hungry, and never feed to the full."[4] "We should take only enough for our needs, otherwise the plants and the animals and the worms we have killed would turn against us and cause us disease and misfortune."[5]

3. Show gratitude for the favor received and always remember the hungry and the starving. This is the moral of invoking or quietly contemplating a blessing before and after eating; a gesture of gratitude and remembrance. A tradition of grace traceable to societies past and present.

   The table manners of Zen monks offer a most elegant example. "As they are arranging the dishes and the waiting monks go around to serve the soup and rice, the Prajna Paramita Hridaya Sutra is recited, followed by the 'Five Meditations' on eating, which are: 'First, of what worth am I? Whence is this offering? Secondly, accepting this offering, I must reflect on the deficiency of my virtue. Thirdly, to guard over my own heart, to keep myself away from faults such as covetousness, etc.—this is the essential thing. Fourthly, this food is taken as good medicine in order to keep the body in a healthy condition. Fifthly, to ensure spiritual attainment, this food is accepted.'. . . They are now ready to take up their chopsticks, but before they actually partake of the sumptuous dinner, the demons or spirits living somewhere in the triple world are remembered; and each monk taking out about seven grains from his own bowl, offers them to those unseen, saying, 'O you, demons and other spiritual beings, I now offer this to you, and may this food fill up the ten quarters of the world and all the demons and other spiritual beings fed therewith.' While eating, quietude prevails. The dishes are handled noiselessly, no word is uttered, no conversation goes on. . . . Nothing is to be left when

4. Hadith of the Prophet Muhammad.
5. Castaneda, *A Separate Reality*, p. 226.

139

the meal is finished. The monks eat up all that is served them, 'gathering up of the fragments that remain.' This is their religion. . . . The tables are now empty as before except those rice grains offered to the spiritual beings at the beginning of the meal. The wooden blocks are clapped, thanks are given, and the monks leave the room in orderly procession as they came in."[6]

4. Back to earth I go when I die to feed worms and vegetation. Ending in a compost heap is a just proposition. Recycled.

5. Given life against overwhelming odds and for sustenance, other creatures—plant or animal—pay dearly. Life must be precious and meant to be worthy and deserving of some praise. I will therefore honor the high promise, preserve life, and pay my dues to the captive creditors whose parts and sum perished so I can survive.

6. All quotations are from D. T. Suzuki, *Essays in Zen Buddhism, First Series* (New York: Grove Press, 1961), pp. 324–25.

Aging: A Concluding Remark

ON THE SUBJECT OF AGING, WE HAVE NO DIFFICULTY finding companionship or enlisting recruits. Obviously, there is a 100-percent participation of readers (and nonreaders). But let us not decay, let us not become sour or turn ugly. Having prepared for aging early on, we can keep our wits, maintain dignity, and renew enthusiasm. We can travel time gracefully and die young as late as possible. Life in all its manifestations is inexhaustible, and it never runs out of thrills, surprises, mystery, and beauty. There is always something worth living for. Said Victor Hugo, "I am now 74, and I am beginning my career." Personally, I have renewed my subscription to Tennessee Williams' profound statement, "Old men were never young." Old age, I expect you (if I am still around), so take your standard time; I will be ready, I promise. No cussing, no fussing. We'll embrace, befriend one another, and keep dancing.

Coping with Handicaps and Disease

The important fact is that when she lost her sight and hearing, she did not lose her mind.

—Ralph Barton Perry[1]

SINCE ADAM AND EVE, DISEASE AND INJURY HAVE been part and parcel of the human condition. An illness or accident of one sort or another is always on the wing, awaiting an opportunity to strike us. At times, the human toll mounts to cataclysmic proportions. Bubonic plague, known as the "Black Death," killed 75 million people in Europe between 1347 and 1351. Baffled and with no good clues to go by, people perceived the pestilence as divine punishment for sin. Non-Christians, the devil's advocate, and perpetrators of evil and wrongdoing were buried alive, with some of the devout uniting in the brotherhood of the flagellants, invoking penance and public whipping to exorcise the menacing tide.

Besieged by the "Black Death" in 1665, distraught Londoners vented their misfortune on dogs and cats, exterminating them in the belief that the poor animals were carriers of the disease. With no cats roaming home and alley, rats had it their way, ate all the food, had all the sex—and their population exploded. The calamitous disease spread like dry forest fire, rapidly consuming the beleaguered inhabitants of the tormented city. Fleas, the real culprit, were given a free ride, happily jumping and deliriously feasting on rats.

Certainly that was not the first time humankind in its blind wrath turned upon a friend, falsely accusing, condemning, and mercilessly penalizing. Predictably, it won't be the last unless

1. Introduction to Helen Keller, *The Story of My Life* (Garden City, N.Y.: Doubleday and Co., 1954), p.16.

we change our modus operandi. At such anguished times, delusion and panic reigned. Syphilis was erroneously thought to confer sorely needed immunity! In all seriousness, many went out of their way to contract the debilitating venereal disease. In 1918–19 the Influenza Pandemic plagued the world, wiping out no less than 50 million people. In those days, the contagious respiratory infection was believed to be a curse from mighty stars of ill fortune. As a result, religious conversions became a panacea, hitting an all-time high.

Over the past few decades, the specific cause and characteristic manifestations of many diseases have been uncovered. Several human ills, deadly before then, became curable. Fatal plague and flu epidemics are now history. Recently, smallpox has been erased from the surface of the earth. For long, its virus brought death and disfigurement to millions. Medical knowledge is now expanding at a fast pace, estimated to double every five years, so that ever increasing breakthroughs are bound to happen.

In the United States, as recently as the 1940s, bacterial infections alone caused 25 percent of all deaths. Today they are responsible for less than 3 percent. The genetic code that governs all our body functions is no more the enigma it used to be. Its detailed structure and the sequence of its components have been clearly deciphered—a momentous achievement having the thrilling potential of unveiling the fundamental causes of the disease process itself. Imagine knowing in conclusive terms why we get sick!

Scientists nowadays foresee gene therapy for diseases currently incurable becoming what antibiotics now are for bacterial infections. Normal genes will then be prescribed and administered to counteract or undo the ill-doings of defective ones. Prenatal detection of genetic disorders as early as the ninth week of pregnancy is currently feasible. A tiny sample of the placenta can be obtained by a relatively simple technique known as chorionic villous sampling, opening up the possibility of in-utero genetic correction before the precious baby is born. Awesome implements to restore, heal, and make well. Exploited, they will import chaos and sorrow.

Right now, despite the immense progress made and the encouraging prospects ahead, in the United States alone more than 42 million people have one or more forms of heart or blood vessel disease; almost one in four adults have high blood pressure; on an annual basis almost 6 million are hospitalized for heart disease; over 2.5 million receive treatment for cancer; nearly 21 million undergo surgery; and 1.5 billion prescription drugs are dispensed. Obviously, we are not as healthy as one might think. A lot remains undone. Incredible as it may sound, we are only just beginning to understand the ABCs of human biology.

Since human diseases and handicaps are not entirely preventable, we ought to know what is available to help us cope. Cancer, traditionally dreaded and considered a death sentence, is survivable 50 percent of the time. Not so grim. Not hopeless. As we saw earlier, excess dietary fat, smoking, and environmental pollutants—all avoidable—make us more vulnerable to cancer. It is estimated that as many as 80 percent of cancers are potentially preventable. Examples include breast self-examination; regular Pap smears; and consulting the physician in the event of irregular bowel habits, lingering constipation, rectal bleeding, continuing cough, difficulty of swallowing, unexplained weight loss or poor appetite, and any other lagging unwell symptoms. Early detection brings early treatment, thereby enhancing the chances of survival.

Timely, appropriate medical management, essential as it is, is but one component in the battle against cancer. The other crucial element is the patient's own attitude and disposition. Those determined not to surrender fight to survive. Wholeheartedly dwelling on the positive, they generally live longer and better, endure less mental and physical anguish, and suffer fewer complications. Their immune system is mobilized against killer cancer cells, curbing their lethal spread, and in some instances providing that pivotal cinch needed to conquer the disease.

144

The following affirmations constitute an important addition to the survival kit of any cancer patient:

I will fight and fight and fight. I am going to make it, I am going to make it. I will survive, I will survive. Licking it, I shall survive. I am wholly determined to kill the cancer before it kills me; yes, yes, I am.

Transformed into action, these maxims do wonders. Verbalizing them frequently and focusing on them in deep concentration with resolute, unshaken conviction are essential. The whole being is stimulated; hope, zest, and cheer come. The doctor and the patient thereby become partners, working together, helping one another toward a common goal. Said the herald: Heal thyself. I hasten to add: With help from the healer.

Killer number one—heart disease—claims nearly 600,000 lives annually in the United States alone. Frightening; yet heart ailments are to a good degree preventable through proper diet, regular exercise, abstinence from smoking, zero to mild alcohol intake, coping with mental stress, early detection and treatment of high blood pressure. All of these are at hand and are realizable with moderate, sincere effort. Medical and surgical treatment for many heart problems is improving, with the outcome better than ever before.

Again, the patient's partnership with the physician can make a difference. Alone, a physician cannot heal; it is a fifty-fifty deal. Generally speaking, patients who are depressed or excessively anxious and tense fare poorly. Heart patient, for the love of life, if you are one of those, *change!* You can! The resources are within you, and nobody should be too proud, too timorous, or too obstinate to seek help when help is needed; and nobody should be so unkind as to deny help to another. Love and compassion heal!

Stroke is a serious malady that every year afflicts a half-million persons in the United States, of whom 150,000 succumb, with many of the survivors disabled in different degrees. In our midst, at any given time, nearly 1 million people are handicapped by this grim disease. Preventive measures for heart disease by and large apply to stroke prevention. In a good number of cases, surgery on the carotid arteries in the neck may prevent strokes.

Fatal kidney damage—much of it, anyway—can be forestalled by curing urinary infections, removing urinary obstructions such as stones or enlarged prostates, and by recognizing and controlling high blood pressure and diabetes. End-stage kidney disease leads to renal failure, known as uremia—a condition once uniformly and rapidly fatal. Now, with the advent of kidney transplantation and dialysis, its outcome has improved, with many victims working, playing, and leading an active life for many years.

Alzheimer's disease is incurable at present, yet its diagnosis should never be presumed by anyone nor made by the unqualified. From 15 to 30 percent of those said to have the disease are in reality suffering mental impairment caused by poor nutrition, infections, unrecognozed injury and other treatable conditions. For families and friends of Alzheimer's patients, the Alzheimer's Disease and Related Disorders Association[2] provides helpful information and access to support groups.

Scientific research promises a solution to the perplexing mystery of this degenerative brain disease. Presently, scientists are focusing on the 21st chromosome (1 of 46 in every human cell). A "marker" of sorts has been located there; 1 gene among 500 encompassed by the chromosome, it may have something to do with the disease. If this is confirmed, the gene (or genes) may then be inoculated in bacterial or animal cell cultures to determine what it does, how, and when. Through genetic engineering, the defective gene may one happy day be rectified or its unwelcome action blocked. Such a happy scenario is by no means certain, not fanciful, either.

Depression and phobias can be reversed by a variety of means: meditation, biofeedback, psychotherapy, and behavioral tech-

2. 70 East Lake Street, Suite 600, Chicago, IL 60601. Tel. (800) 621–0379.

niques. Carefully selected drugs are helpful in some instances. There is no acceptable reason for being wracked by fear or diminished by depression. Search for help. It *is* available.

Chemical dependency on alcohol and other drugs has increasingly become a matter of national concern—a shame and a nightmare. It is widespread among all social strata, regardless of income level and educational background. As a matter of necessity, the intellect/psyche of our nation must be cleansed of these most hazardous pollutants. It is urgent. Everyone stands to gain—abuser and abused, the latter embracing families, friends, community, and the country at large. Withdrawal symptoms can be frightfully mean and sometimes unendurable, requiring hospitalization. Community hospitals have doubled the number of their inpatient and outpatient chemical dependency units between 1980 and 1985. Good results make the undertaking worthwhile.

AIDS (*a*cquired *i*mmuno*d*eficiency *s*yndrome) is a fatal condition, yet slowly and piecemeal we are learning more and more about the elusive virus that triggers a chain reaction consuming body organs and tissues. Despite the gloom above and ahead of us, a breakthrough will dawn. Despair, apathy and hostility will not cure AIDS. With no remedy on hand, preventive measures are now the only shield we have for combat.

These include: sex education before adolescence; avoiding anal intercourse and multiple sex partners; the use of condoms; total abstinence from intravenous drugs; screening blood donors for the virus; and transfusing blood and blood products only when absolutely necessary. Whenever possible, if major surgery is anticipated, timely provision should be made for one's own blood to be drawn, safely stored, and transfused as needed during and after surgery. This process, called autotransfusion, is worth considering and talking over with your physician. For information and referral to local AIDS projects and clinics, call the Center for Disease Control Hotline (800) 447–AIDS or the National Gay Task Force (800) 221-7044.

Chronic pain may grow intolerably nagging and debilitating.

If the cause cannot be identified and eliminated, several methods to ameliorate its severity ought to be sought, such as physical therapy, rehabilitation, psychotherapy, acupuncture, and special local and regional anesthetic techniques. Nationwide, most medical centers have comprehensive pain centers or clinics. Valuable information can be obtained by writing to the National Chronic Pain Outreach Association, 8222 Wycliffe Court, Manassas, VA 22110.

Diabetes to a large extent is a disease of opulence and satiety. One of every twenty Americans is diabetic. The cornerstone of treatment is still dietetic under medical supervision; however, oral drugs may become necessary to control the disease. For the large number of diabetics who need daily insulin injections, the good word is that oral insulin is on the horizon, and an implantable artificial pancreas is in the offing. The clever implant senses the patient's blood sugar level and infuses insulin accordingly. This feature eliminates the danger of over- or under-dosage of insulin.

An artificial arm and hand unit with practical dexterity was developed at the University of Utah in 1981. The unit is controlled by electrodes and a microprocessor that responds to brain messages sent through the remaining shoulder and arm muscles. The ingenious device has been fitted on several hundred people worldwide. A skillful three-finger, one-thumb robot hand will be ready in the very near future. For several years, irreparably damaged hips, knees, and finger joints have been replaced by artificial ones with gratifying long-term results, making it possible for many to walk, work, write, and dance.

Have you ever wondered how many Americans are hearing-impaired? Believe it or not, up to 20 million, with about 2 million of these being profoundly deaf. Hearing aids have now reached an acme of sophistication: the latest ones can be surgically implanted, are less visible, and deliver a better quality of sound. Microscopic surgery permits reconstruction of the ear drum and the tiny, delicate bones that transmit sound. In certain cases where hearing aids are not helpful, there is yet another answer. An electronic ear known as the cochlear implant has recently broken the barrier of deafness. If all fails, the manual signs and gestures of time-honored sign language can be effectively used to communicate thoughts and ideas, carrying on conversations as well.

Glaucoma—a leading cause of blindness—is treatable, thanks to newer drugs administered in the form of eyedrops. In cases not well controlled by medication alone, eye surgery, including the use of laser, is fairly safe and quite efficient in lowering the eyeball pressure.

Blind people have been reading books by Braille for many years, but of the more than 50,000 books published annually in the United States, fewer than 500 are transcribed into Braille. New and thrilling things are happening now. A reading machine for the blind has been in use since 1976. Simple to operate, the blind person places the printed material on a glass-topped optical scanner which will read aloud in sing-song voice about 200 words a minute. The machine is programmed to give some stress and pauses in order to make sentences more intelligible. It can be slowed down by the listener and even made to spell out difficult or incomprehensible words.[3] The machine is usually found in libraries, schools, and companies and government agencies employing the blind.

Compact portable reading machines convert printed text either into tactile letters felt by the fingertips or into audible speech. One blind airline reservationist processes more than 80 calls with her portable optical, exceeding the volume handled by her sighted colleagues.

The Talking Books Program is of immense value and of no cost to the beneficiary. The local community library, as an agent for the Library of Congress, provides a simple tape player and a special record player designed to run at very slow speeds. A world of books and a selection from a large variety of other

3. Kurzwell's Reading Machine, 33 Cambridge Parkway, Cambridge, MA 02142.

literature and magazines are read in a warm, highly professional manner. Now, electronic editing of Braille offers paperless Braille systems to the blind, and with it a whole array of computer systems has come within reach.[4]

With loss of vision, deterioration happens not only to space perception but also to that of time. At the push of a button, a variety of Talking Clocks[5] tell the blind the exact time of day or night. The faithful Seeing Eye dog has for so long been safely guiding the blind and never goes out of fashion. The electronic equivalent of the Seeing Eye dog has recently been built: a proficient sonar device.

A large number of people have severely impaired vision or are legally blind. Closed-circuit television (CCTV) systems give electronic magnification, allowing many of these people to continue working as teachers, judges, attorneys, and clerks. Their leisure activities can also be secured. High-powered spectacles with "honeybee" lenses are among several simple tools available to assist the 1.5 million legally blind in the United States. Victims of stroke, cerebral palsy, and a host of other conditions often have severe speech defects. Phonetically based synthesizers with touch-sensitive switches allow them to communicate effectively with others.

---

4. VersaBraille by Telesensory Systems, Inc.; Microbrailler from Triformation Systems Inc.; and the Braille Display Processor from V-Tek, Inc.
5. Manufactured by the Sharp Corporation.

Helen Keller, C. H. Fowler, and
Michael Naranjo

RECALLING HIS MEMORABLE STUDENT'S SENIOR YEAR
at Radcliffe College, Ralph Barton Perry wrote, "When you
communicate with her, you know you have reached her 'inner ear' and the 'eye of her mind'; which is more than can
be said of most so-called conversations among those whose
external hearing and vision are unimpaired."[1] Perry was refer-
ring to Helen Keller, who took a course with Perry in outlines
of the history of philosophy at Harvard.

At the tender age of 19 months, Helen, of Tuscumbia, Ala-
bama, was destined to endure. A grave illness struck, leaving
her deaf, blind, and mute—a cruel blow. For the rest of her
life, Helen had but touch, smell, and taste to sample the world
and reach others—three receptors, imprecise and limited in
range.

On the advice of Alexander Bell,[2] her parents employed a
teacher from the Perkins School of the Blind in Boston. Helen
was six when Ann Mansfield Sullivan left Boston for the Kellers'
mansion. Annie herself was not a routine presence; rather a
personne extraordinaire, she was 20 years old then, partially
blind, delicately built, but not fragile. Her exterior air of cold
remoteness was tempered by the endearing leer of a cherry
blossom. Like a kitten given new surroundings, Annie was
timorous and brash, yet the experienced eye could tell that her
soft paws were shielding sharp claws. Her core was fortitude,
yet never failing to yield or opt for friendship and compassion.
She could make things happen and could produce miracles

---

1. Introduction to Helen Keller, *The Story of My Life* (Garden City, N.Y.:
Doubleday and Co., 1954), p. 17.
2. Alexander Graham Bell (1847–1922), inventor of the telephone, was
an authority on speech correction and the teaching of speech to the deaf.

when miracles were least expected or hopelessly hoped for. Touching Helen's feeling hand to the doll, Annie then pressed "D–O–L–L" onto Helen's palm, thereby teaching the child the names of objects. "Eighteen nouns and three verbs—they're in her fingers now; I need only time to push one of them into her mind! One, and everything under the sun will follow."[3]

Overcoming Helen's tantrums and refusing to accept or be intimidated by the Kellers' parental protection and unrestrained pity for their handicapped, spoiled child, Annie could then win an unwinnable battle. Two years later, Helen could read and write in Braille. At age nine, she spoke those miraculous words: *"I am not dumb now."* Touching her fingers to Annie's larynx to "hear" the vibrations, she was able to speak. Her voice was not generally intelligible; still, she toured the world with the help of a translator, promoting education of the deaf and the blind.

At this time on my writing desk stand some books and two paintings by Ted De Grazia: *Niños con Flores* and *The Pink Bird. Warm Day in Autumn* gracefully occupies a corner of the cluttered desk. Mouth-painted by C. H. Fowler, the picture and I often relate to one another, and through our intimate dialogues, we became friends. I carry this warm scene in the art gallery of my mind, where, in solitude, I can contemplate and review at my pleasure. An insubstantial river marches on, seemingly certain of its course—gentle, low ripples telling of the smooth ride and playing to my mind's ear the everlasting melody of water current flowing, roaring serene and mild.

How sweet, how comforting! All familiar, all beautiful—and I am so happy. Well . . . equilibrated would be more like it. Rivers meet bridges and run underneath. Fowler's bridge permits the river to pass on, while above is an artist-painted rendezvous between two unnamed lovers. My admiring eye revels

3. William Gibson, *The Miracle Worker, A Play* (New York: Samuel French, 1956), p. 79 (1985 edition).

in the artist's creation of the loving affection with which the two strangers behold one another. I can tell: the two will remain bridge-bound, spell-bound, autumn-bound.

In the bridge's vicinity stand two trees conveying a vague sense. Sadness is it? Or could it be that, in their secretive state of anticipation, a pensive mood surfaced? Can plants anticipate, hope, be sad, or become pensive? I have no way of telling, yet from what I see, both trees took their autumn call and I, the observer, can't help anticipating the promised spring coming on time with its perennial gift of good weather, youthful looks, new leaves, new birds, new thrills.

Other trees in the picture—slower and thriftier, perhaps wiser—still hold on to their autumn leaves; their spread of yellow, brown, orange, and varying shades of red still recites the poignant poems of autumn. Eventually, the season must play its final tune, reminding those pretty, lingering leaves that they must come down, that new leaves are on the threshold to inherit time and place on the twigs of their beloved tree.

With every whiff of the autumn breeze, the playful grass on the river banks dances and dances, and this friendly rustle readily lays hold of me, so that here I am, dancing, dancing—merrily, effortlessly, lightheartedly, just like the tall grass on the banks of the river. The river is now getting smaller, and finally it vanishes beyond the lovers' bridge. What goes on thereafter? The picture doesn't tell. Fleeing the down-road of lamentation and self-pity, C. H. Fowler's undaunted spirit lifts us up high, along with her, to a warm, joyful plateau. Fowler, her mouth-held brush, *Warm Day in Autumn*, and myself are in a certain sense one.

"It may sound strange, but I don't even think about being handicapped and I haven't for a long time. . . . Instead, I thank God I'm alive—and concentrate on my work." Michael Naranjo, a Tewa Indian from a Pueblo Reservation in New Mexico, lost his eyesight and the use of his right hand in Vietnam as a result of a grenade explosion on January 8, 1968. He went back to working with clay and then on to making bronze sculptures. His bronze sculpture *The Secret* is beautiful and philosophical. It tells of an old man who raised a crow that lives in a nearby tree. Every time the old man goes for a stroll, the crow flies to his shoulder and whispers secrets in his left ear. In 1972, President and Mrs. Nixon invited him to show his sculptures at the White House, and in 1983, at the request of Pope John Paul II, Naranjo exhibited his work at the Vatican.

No matter what the odds are, despite the handicaps and the letdowns, there is always a way. In this world, nothing is permanent. Everything, every condition, every event is subject to change. Why ever concede final defeat? Why surrender hope? You are defeated and your situation is hopeless because you think so and believe it. Such an attitude goes against the nature of things, against the very nature of life itself. An alternative always exists. Find it, take it, work with it.

Coping with Stress:
A Personal Experience

THE STRESS YOU AND I HAVE BEEN EXPERIENCING from time to time is our own product, and the difficulties we have been encountering in coping with it are all negotiable and surmountable. Inasmuch as we are the makers, unmake it we can, undo it we must. Stress is one's own reaction to a perceived misfortune or to an unwelcome or threatening expectation. The response largely depends on one's own perception of the events. Stress is merely a warning signal telling that something has gone wrong, is going wrong, or will soon go wrong.

Viewed as such, stress becomes an eye-opener, useful, physiologic and positive. What ultimately counts is what we do next. Taken as an end in itself, stress turns into a troublesome dilemma, a mouse-trap generating nothing but frustration, neurosis, insomnia, appetite loss, unexplained fatigue, serious physical ailments, binges, and depression. Eventually this self-fostered adversary does away with the simple joys of life. Finally, the instinctive desire to live may die out. The path is bleak, one of self-destruction, often extending to the destruction of others as well.

It is absolutely necessary to comprehend stress and to see it as it is, without misconceptions. Equally important is not to accept it as an article of fate or a judgment dictated by circumstances beyond our control. Stress is not final, is not predetermined, is not irreversible.

When I am all right, I am adjusted and I know it: a state of evenness of mind and calm composure. I take notice of the sunrise, look at the flowers and consciously acknowledge their presence and experience their loveliness, listen to the birds and watch their gay flight, feel and endorse everything I touch, enjoy and appreciate my early-morning hot shower, shave without cutting the wrinkles on my cheeks or bruising the furrow beneath my underlip, drive to work without getting incensed by other motorists' indiscretions and keeping in mind not to insist on the right of way.

I perform my work with serenity, sincerity, enthusiasm, and inward contentment. I eat to no excess, in no rush, while affirming the taste of my food before swallowing it, and expressing gratitude for the nourishment received. When going to bed, I fall asleep without alcohol or sleeping pills. I wake up in the morning, fresh, relaxed, with renewed hope and eager commitment to have a good day and help others have a good day, or at the very least not to obstruct their pursuit of happiness. What it all means is that I am concentrating, doing my best, and living in the present tense, besides keeping a good rapport with others, circumstances, time, environment and accepting the world as it is.

I can't claim that every day all goes well and dandy. No, no. Ugly banners; writing on the wall spelling threat and danger; bad news; betrayal by friends; uncalled-for malice from associates trusted and admired; backbiting; losses on the job; opportunities sweet and cozy flying away just when I am about ready to harvest them, ending in the undeserving laps of some others; sickness, personal or afflicting family or friends. Of all these "goodies," I think I'm getting my share, more or less. Like many, I conveniently have others to blame; culprits of sorts, they do me in. And it hurts.

Granted, all of this or even more may be true; but I must admit: I am not pure and innocent either. Knowingly and unknowingly I must have stepped on some toes. Simply stated, my gain is someone else's loss, and it is natural for humans to react hastily and angrily to their loss. Ignoring others, hurting their pride, and paying little or no regard to their feelings —more than likely I have done some of those awful things. In short, and in all fairness, quite a bit of what I get—good or bad—is self-instigated. I don't doubt it for a moment.

This may sound moralistic and confessional, and on the surface it may also seem a far cry from the subject of coping with stress. On the contrary, here it belongs, a legitimate part of the subject matter. A considerable degree of our stress is bitching and moaning about the raw deal we believe we are getting from co-workers, neighbors, and loved ones in return for our noble deeds and acts of charity. A substantial portion is anger at God—or fate—for placing us at the bottom of the totem pole and ruthlessly kicking us down whenever we manage to climb up the ladder. *Why me!* is a familiar cry of protest exuding dissatisfaction and sorrow. This web of misconception must be dismantled if we are to rid ourselves of a major cause of stress, namely the illusion of undeserved suffering.

So, Suggestion Number One: *When what you consider misfortune hits your door, before pointing an accusing finger at others or at heaven, sincerely try to find out what went wrong, take a good look, courageously allocate your share and accept responsibility. Work at changing things and rectifying errors. Lamentation and self-pity will only make things worse and hand you over to the unkind state of prolonged stress, which breeds mental and physical illness.*

Be your own analyst, therapist, and best friend. Nobody knows you better or is likely to love you more. We owe it to ourselves to recognize stress early on before it takes root and mushrooms within our fertile pulp. The signs are all too obvious and easy to reckon. Here are some common examples: cursing when the alarm clock wakes you up; habitual urge for a drink before leaving for work; frequently yelling at your spouse, kids, or roommate; ignoring your faithful, loving dog or your purring cat, its silky fur softly touching your legs with no approbation or affectionate response on your part; not noticing the sun or the clouds hiding the sun; eyes blind to flowers, grass, and trees; ears deaf to the keynote of nature, the rustle of tree leaves, birds' talk, the sound of rainfall and music; cussing when rush hour traffic slows you down; slamming doors and windows; huffing, puffing, and fussing while handling routine matters; inability to concentrate; smoking one cigarette after another; drinking coffee cup after cup; unexplainable fatigue; insomnia; being hooked on booze; dependency on sleeping pills; affinity to tranquilizers; frequent visitation by terrible dreams.

Contrary to common belief, major problems end up having simple solutions. It may sound paradoxical—yet it is utterly true. We are taken by the froth, the smoke, the siren and commotion filling the air. We run after each, trying hard to decipher the multiple outward manifestations. The search goes on, the road stretches on, trails diverge, confusion grows, frustration mounts. Stress feeds and thrives on such a state of affairs; all at the expense of its busy host: *us*.

So, Suggestion Number Two: *There are no problems without solutions. Those problems that appear unsolvable will cease to be. They don't exist, never did in the first place. Problems come with their solutions. Both interlocked, each is dependent on the other and cannot be without it. A world full of problems and nothing but problems is a figment of the confused, the pessimistic, and the cynical. The world can't go around propelled and charged with problems alone. Such a world will soon go off track and tumble down. The world's balance rests on twin pillars: problems and corresponding solutions.*

Humankind for the most part keeps breathlessly racing between the two extremes, not seeing or accepting both. Those seeing nothing but solutions, rainbows, rose gardens, bounty, and joy are enchanted fools. Those exclusively seeing problems with endless pain, sorrow, loss, and tears are miserable souls living doomsday and experiencing a dismal abyss. The few who see the two halves of the world, the two sides of the coin, are wise and secure, at peace with themselves and the world, ever affluent, their capital consisting of right seeing, good thought, and a high spirit.

Suggestion Number Three: *If and when you get what you want, enjoy it! Remember, most of us neglect or fail to take pleasure in and use with satisfaction what we have worked so diligently to achieve. Hastening on to another pursuit without a pause is foolhardy and stressful. Pause for poise and repose.*

Suggestion Number Four: *If and when you get what you want, don't get carried away and don't count on a repeat. The fruits of your labor are due in part to your own good effort and in some degree to a combination of favorable conditions not wholly subject to your control. Be thankful, humble, and gracious when you succeed; don't grieve when you fail. Remember: to the loser belong some spoils; and calamity often lurks under the wings of victory.*

Suggestion Number Five: *"What has happened has happened; what has gone is gone. If only one understands this, there is nothing to suffer from."*[1]

Suggestion Number Six: *We cannot predict the future. Logic is not enough, intellect cannot do it, and intuition cannot always be right. Knowing the future isn't all that good anyway. If we do, we shall lose anticipation, enthusiasm, and choice. Foreknowledge, besides being impossible, will make our world dull and confining.*

1. Katsuki Sekida, *Zen Training* (New York: Weatherhill, 1975), p. 104.

Down-to-Earth Guidelines I Found Effective in Coping with My Own Stress

Knowing, understanding, and believing the foregoing six suggestions.

Naturally, belief is most important. Knowledge is easier to acquire, understanding less easy. Belief is strictly a personal matter and might dawn gradually or suddenly. True, there is a whole stack of beliefs deeply rooted in almost everyone's consciousness. Many of them defy understanding and remain immune to logic and rationality, but in coping with a problem of some magnitude such as stress, understanding boosts belief, thereby enhancing the condition of the believer and making him or her better qualified to help others trapped in the same predicament.

Practicing what we believe in.

Belief without practice will not turn things around and won't solve problems. Practice without belief in what we do is short-lived. Sooner or later the individual will lose heart and go back to old habit and routine, and so on to the joyless ride again and again. Belief keeps us right on track, committed and sincere. Belief breeds life into our endeavors.

Daily doses of slowing down.

A most important remedy. Whatever we have gained through speed, valuable and splendid as it may seem, we have lost more to restlessness and anxiety generated by the sustained fast pace. Pauses to enjoy and recollect are essential if the human organs and systems are to recover. The wear and tear of speed are awesome. Effective methods of slowing down are discussed in earlier pages in this book.

Suffice it to restate that walking and meditation have been effective in neutralizing and mending the harm speed inflicts on our systems. Sports and hobbies fall into this category; true, some have a quick pace, but this is a horse of a different color. Extracurricular pursuits open other avenues, help us see more, hear better, feel deeper, while keeping our mind interested and our body fit.

Not being limited by a rigid set of goals.
When things come to a dead end, change strategy. If the new approach takes you to the same place, adopt new goals. Fixation and clinging to objects—goals included—is stressful and frequently disappointing. Personally, I have learned this one the hard way! The wise have goals as well, but to them the path and the goal are one and the same, so they remain free of worry and anxiety. For the elect few, the goal is infinite. If our goal becomes infinite, we will forfeit the treadmill mentality, the sense of rush, the attitude of urgency, and the spirit of combat. Energy then renews itself and never runs out. This is likened to "second wind," which imparts ease and a recovered capacity for continuing any kind of endeavor.

These guidelines are my closing statement. On many levels, you know what I am talking about, what I have tried to convey. Now: the silence that accompanies *being it*.

> *Wisdom ripens into silence,*
> *And the lesson she does teach*
> *Is that life is more than language*
> *And that thought is more than speech.*